# ELEVATE YOUR HEALTH

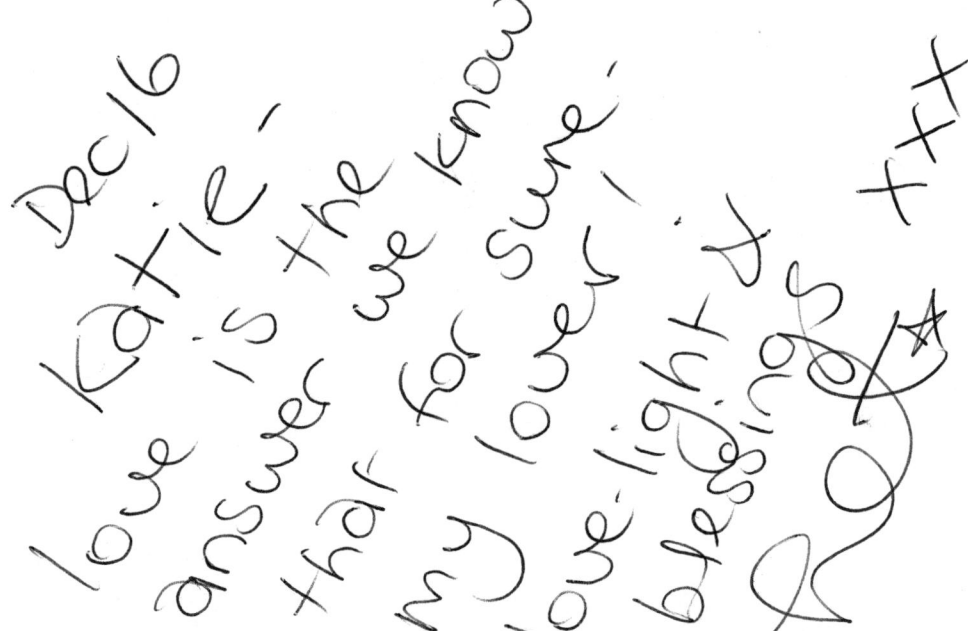

Dec 16
Katie -
love is the know
answer we know
that for sure -
my lover !
love-light &
blessings xxx

# ELEVATE YOUR HEALTH

THE MOST INSPIRING WAY TO TAKE YOUR HEALTH TO THE NEXT LEVEL

**Foreword by Dr John Demartini**
Human Behaviour Specialist, Educator & Teacher From "The Secret"

**Disclaimer**

All the information, techniques, skills and concepts contained within this publication are of the nature of general comment only and are not in any way recommended as individual advice. The intent is to offer a variety of information to provide a wider range of choices now and in the future, recognising that we all have widely diverse circumstances and viewpoints.

Should any reader choose to make use of the information contained herein, this is their decision, and the contributors (and their companies), authors and publishers do not assume any responsibilities whatsoever under any condition or circumstances. It is recommended that the reader obtain their own independent advice.

First Edition 2016

National Library of Australia

Cataloguing-in-Publication entry:

Creator: Harvey, Benjamin J., author.

Other Authors:

Chhabra, Shivi | Edge, Jennifer | Frawley, Maree | Gangaram, Ameeta | Genovese, Antonietta | Johnson, Ruby | Jukes, Suzy | Koelman, Anke | Murphy, Heather Belle | Printziou, Catherine | Salmon, Libby | Williams, Russell

Title: Elevate Your Health / Benjamin J Harvey.

ISBN: 9781925471021 (paperback)

Series: Elevate books.

Subjects:
Health.
Well-being.

Dewey Number: 613

Published by Author Express
From Inspiration to Publication in 5 Simple Steps
www.AuthorExpress.com
publish@authorexpress.com

# Dedication

*To fellow learners wanting to take
their health to the next level.
This book is dedicated to you.*

**Benjamin J Harvey and co-authors**

# Foreword by Dr John Demartini

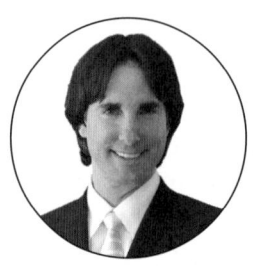

For over forty years, I've studied the art of wellness and the healing arts, particularly in relation to the mind-body connection. I have a background as a chiropractor, and I study the integration of psychology and philosophy.

In particular I've been involved in axiology, which is the study of worth and values. Every human being lives by a hierarchy of values, and no two people have the same ones. People's values, or priorities, are as unique to that individual as their fingerprints or eye retina. Because of this, people filter the world through their values and perceive situations.

Something that's of highest value is what you're inspired from within to do. No one needs to remind you to get up in the morning. You love doing it. On the other hand, you procrastinate on the lowest values and require outside motivation.

The hierarchy of these values also affects your physiology. In other words, how the body functions. How you perceive the world according to your values affects your cells, genetics and physical condition.

There's an underlying psychology of health conditions people have in their everyday lives. The body shows you signs and symptoms as feedback to point you in the direction and guide you to be your most congruent, authentic and inspired self in order to live your most fulfilled life. Basically, if you're not living according to your highest values, you're low on energy and have illness in the body. Hate and anger can run down the immune system. It's a well-known fact that anger, loss and stress can lead to cancer. Unbalanced emotions will lead to illness, and love and appreciation will lead you back to wellness.

Vitality in life is proportionate to your vision. You're in the highest vibration when you're living your authentic life. When you live according to your highest values, you're rewarded physiologically with increased energy.

Throughout this book you will find healers with various methodologies, all ultimately working to bring your body back to homeostasis. A therapist or healer who works from a space of love and gratitude of the heart and certainty and presence of mind, will affect a healing in anyone with whom he/she comes into contact. There's absolutely a place for their healing modalities and treatments, though it's important to realise that all true wellness starts in the mind and works through the heart.

In terms of health, I believe everyone should eat to live and not live to eat. Drink lots of water, and be grateful.

You can be a master of your destiny or a victim of your history. When you go to bed with gratitude, you wake up with inspiration. I'm certain that practicing gratitude will *Elevate Your Health*.

What I know for sure is that gratitude causes your heart to open and for love to flow, and love is the greatest healer in life.

**Dr John F. Demartini**
Human Behaviour Specialist, Educator & Teacher From "The Secret"
www.DrDemartini.com

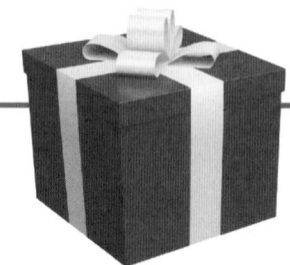

# BONUS GIFT

# The Elevate YOU
## 7 Day Transformation

## Want to take the top 7 areas of your life to the next level?

There is ONE powerful 'Elevate Process' you can use immediately to improve Your Relationships, Health, Finances, Mindset and any other area of your life.

In this transformational 7 day online course, Benjamin J Harvey guides you through the "Elevate Process" and how you can improve your life from the inside-out.

**Normally valued at $295**
**Get FREE and instant access here:**

## www.elevate-books.com/you

Life Rewards Action. Get started today!

# Contents

"Giving yourself permission
to do what you love is the key to
elevating all areas of your life."

*~ Benjamin J Harvey*

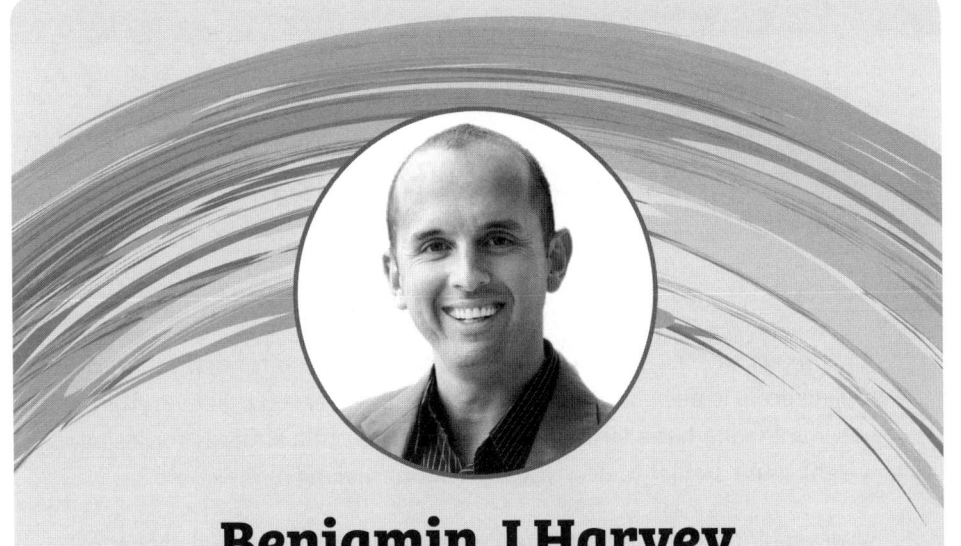

# Benjamin J Harvey

## Heal Your Health

In his pursuit to assist people in finding the answers to life's most intriguing questions, Benjamin J Harvey has studied the psychology of empowerment for over ten years. Knowing that reading books like the Elevate series empowers people to bring their dreams into reality, Benjamin has been assisting thousands of people across the globe to empower themselves and live abundantly on purpose.

In 2009 he founded Authentic Education with business partner Cham Tang, to help empower people to live abundantly on purpose. As a result, Authentic Education went on to achieve something that has never been done before in the history of personal development. They received the BRW Fast Starters Award in 2013 and then backed it up in 2015 by being named in the BRW Fast 100 as the thirty-eigth fastest-growing company in Australia.

# Benjamin J Harvey

## Heal Your Health

All humans have a common a desire to feel good and for many, part of feeling good is being at their ideal weight. I've learned that everything you want in life has a strategy, so I've worked out a strategy for losing weight that's similar to how you'd go about making money.

At one point in my life I achieved what I call the debt-to-weight ratio. My 130kg weight matched my financial debt, which was over $130,000. I've since lost the excess weight and paid off the debt, and now I'm devoting this chapter to helping you achieve your health goals.

**Why do you think you became overweight?**

I think the key reason I became overweight was a combination of depression and the amount of medication I was taking for the depression. I believe that has an impact on the body's ability to digest food correctly and burn fuel.

**How long did it take you to achieve the weight loss, and what did you consider the main factor behind it?**

To actually lose the weight it took me six months or so, and this was after making a commitment that it was time to change it all around. The only thing is, I didn't consciously say, "I'm going to lose weight", so I didn't go out of my way to do it. What I did was just fall in love with myself and do more inner work. Personal development.

I wasn't satisfied with my weight, and I was kind of embarrassed and pretty ashamed of how I looked, but I wasn't getting up in the mornings saying I needed to love myself. So the key distinction to me was that when I corrected my inner world and was able to get on track and start becoming friends with myself, I was able to change the way I ate, the way I digested and the way I operated, which resulted in the weight vanishing off of my body that I've now kept off for fourteen years.

**What was the motivation for you to start your weight loss journey?**

The core motivation for me was a deeper desire to find who I truly was. I had a deeper desire to fix what I classed as a "broken" mind, so for me it wasn't just a weight thing. I didn't buy magazines and dream of this fit body or imagine myself at the beach with a six pack. I just imagined what it might be like waking up one day and realising I didn't hate myself and not having suicidal thoughts. It was a journey of figuring out if I was normal or permanently broken, because so many people convinced me I was broken. I wanted to discover if I could fix my mind.

The motivation really was always around the internal world of becoming happy and feeling normal. I guess it was a desire for...enlightenment, for lack of a better term, and real self-love without all of the shame and guilt.

**What fears did you have to overcome at the start of that journey?**

Trying to identify who I would be without the thoughts. I've had issues throughout my life, right back to when I was six years of age, when I first had a major trauma take place. Ever since then I'd always had some form of issue or noise inside of my mind; an internal mental chatter.

With Authentic Education, and working with thousands of individuals a year, we've discovered that even though people will say spiders or public speaking is a big fear, change is really the number one, because there are parts of the hindbrain that are designed to keep you alive and protect you. If you change into someone new, or you change something in your life, your hindbrain deems that as uncertainty and therefore doesn't know whether or not it can protect you.

So there's a primordial instinct in your body when you want to change that can prevent you from achieving it. Therefore, I'd have to say my biggest fear was just more of a primordial bodily function of not knowing who I would be if I didn't have these issues and how I would relate to the world if I didn't always have a problem inside of my mind. There was an inner fear of wondering if I'd like the person I became once I remove all of this other stuff.

**Did you start alone or with support?**

I had a lot of support around me, but there is a quote that says:

> "It's not that we know so much,
> it's that we know so much that isn't so."

I went and saw a lot of these so-called experts who had all of these amazing opinions about how you're meant to make yourself better, and one of them convinced me that for the rest of my life I would have to eat Lithium pills and get blood tests to check my Lithium levels. For some reason, I believed this person for at least a good five years. So from 1997 to 2002 I would take handfuls of Lithium every day, as well as other forms medication such as Zyprexas and Olanzapine. I also had to take small doses of Valium as well.

What I learned is that the people I spoke with were giving me information based on their model of the world. Their solutions were focussed on what they'd studied at university or what they read in their own articles they chose to refer to. As a result, they had only one approach for helping people. So, I'd go and see a counsellor, and they'd give me a counselling approach. I'd go see a psychologist, and they'd give me a psychological approach. I'd go and see a psychiatrist, and they gave me a psychiatric approach.

Back in 1997, I was as skinny as a rail, unhealthily so, because I wasn't eating food at all. After many, many years of battling with my own depression and taking all of this medication, my weight began to fluctuate. It was a strange journey. My body had gone through such extremes, and it wasn't until later that I realised once you've been given all of the best advice in the world, the next step is to do it on your own. At the end of the day, people know their body. It really is your best friend if you learn to listen to it. Your body will tell you a whole range of important information if you're present enough to be able to hear what it's saying. So after getting all of the best advice I could, I don't use any of it today.

I decided it was probably time to listen to myself. As a result, I changed a lot in my life, like for instance my medication intake. In fact by 2002 I'd stopped all forms of medication, not because some psychiatrist told me to, but because it didn't seem right to me. Then I stopped reliving my past and telling everybody about it, which is what psychologists were trying to get me to do.

I guess at some point you have to back yourself and listen to your own intuition. This is when it becomes important to realise that deep down inside, you do want the best for yourself.

**What challenges have you experienced in life, and how have you overcome them and/or continue to overcome them today?**

I think at the end of the day it has to do with a saying inscribed by a Delphic oracle on the pronaos, which is the forecourt of the temple of Apollo, and later made famous by Aristotle and Plato: *know thyself.* The most important lesson I've learned is that every challenge that's come my way has been feedback to get myself to learn a little bit more about who I am at the deepest level.

I've discovered that people generally sabotage themselves in three specific ways,

1.  Money

2.  Relationships

3.  Health

So if you find that you're getting negative feedback in any one of those areas, understand you're getting a signal that you're not getting to know yourself enough, and also that you're not giving yourself permission to fall in love with that person you're getting to know.

For me, the single biggest challenge I've ever experienced in life was the ability to get over some major abuse that happened when I was a kid. To move past the shame and guilt and still be able to look into the mirror and say that I love myself. There's a saying in the personal development industry that says you're only as sick as your secrets, and I find that a lot of weight issues have to do with people keeping secrets deep down inside they're so ashamed of and feel guilty about. But rather than expressing those out to the world for the purposes of healing, they consume food as a way of equilibrating the emotional charges.

Everybody's trying to self-medicate in some way, shape or form. Some use gambling, some use medication, some use drugs or alcohol, and some people use food. When they eat, it gives them a specific type of feeling that helps to counterbalance or override the deepest shame and guilt that's really going on for them.

When people use food as a way of self-medicating in order to get over deep shame and guilt or fears, that craving momentarily takes their attention off the bigger issue. Those who continually or constantly eat and gain weight are really attempting to find a process of medicating themselves.

### What important lesson have you learnt from your experience?

This is going to sound really clichéd. If you look back through history at all of the different mystics and gurus in the world of transformation, most agree you have to be childlike and playful, and a common phrase they use is that you must do what you love. So if there was anything I've learnt along my journey is not to take life too seriously. As Oscar Wilde wisely pointed out, "Life is too important to be taken seriously", and I tend to agree with that statement.

I think people need to take it easy and enjoy the ride. If you don't take yourself lightly, you're going to be heavy all of your life, so you need to lighten up a little bit. It's all a big game, and we're here to have fun and experience as much love as possible. The better you play the game the more love you can experience, and that's kind of the reward for knowing you're playing the game correctly.

If you're sitting around all day long, overeating and sleeping on the couch, lethargic from all of the food you're eating, you're going to be drained and tired and sleepy all of the time anyway and won't have time to do what you love. It winds up being a catch-22. Do you find the time to do what you love before you love yourself? Or do you love yourself and then go and do what you love? I don't have the answer as to which one comes first, but what I do know is that you can't have one without the other. A lot of people are battling with weight issues because of a lack of self-love and self-worth.

Fundamentally, if people want to start losing weight they need to start doing what they love. Obviously you have to do the mindset work as well and deal with whatever shame and guilt is underneath the surface, but a great first step would be to make one list of everything you love and another of what you do daily, and then adjust accordingly until both lists pretty much line up with each other. Then you're good to go.

Be childlike and playful and at all cost, make sure you do what you love.

**What challenges have you faced keeping the weight off once you lost it, and how have you overcome them?**

The challenge when you've gained a lot of weight is that you've expanded, excuse the pun, not just your waistline but your parameters past the point that's acceptable for your body to grow. For me it's a matter of setting a brand-new set of rules. I have guidelines inside of my mind that say, *No worries. You can go well over a hundred kilos. You've done it before*, and I have parameters that say, *Yeah, you can go way less than sixty-five kilos. You've done it before.*

Now when I weigh less than sixty-five kilos, I really do look terribly ill because of the way my face goes so gaunt, and it looks like I'm literally starving myself to death. And certainly when I go up to the ninety five and above, I start to look a lot like the Michelin man, so I had to reset my parameters.

I had to have a system of knowing what the acceptable buffer zone was for me to fit within, and once I figured it out I just had to reset the idea inside my mind. Doing what I love and having a bit of a plan got the weight off. I think people do need an eating plan. It's important to have a default eating strategy. This way if you find you're getting lost in life and don't know what's going on, and you get on the scales and realise you've gained weight, you have a master reset button like the kind that used to be at the bottom of old toys.

I don't tell too many people about this, but inside my phone I have a default eating plan. This way any time I feel like I'm binging or consuming too many foods, I pull out my default eating plan and drive straight to the shops to buy everything on the shopping list that provides me food for a week. I follow this up by making sure there's nothing in my house that's going to affect my success. Then for an entire week I just eat this plan.

Now, this plan is one that's used by natural body builders as a way to trim down before competitions. It's not in any way, shape or form a diet, because you eat so much food it's ridiculous. In fact, it's even more food than I would normally eat, but because of the combinations of foods and the frequency with which you eat them, it definitely does have a metabolic effect on the body and activates a trim-down function. My brother does a lot of body building, so he often will share with me different strategies around how to trim down. I'd say I use it maybe once every two years, if that.

I think people do forget to stick to their eating plan sometimes. So if you find yourself doing things the old way, don't beat yourself up about it and get annoyed, upset or guilty. Like if I showed you a shortcut to work after you'd been driving the same way there for fifty years, maybe two or three months afterward you might forget the shortcut and drive the old way to work. Instead of getting upset with yourself, have a giggle about it and just get back on track.

There's a saying in body building that says you can't out-train a bad diet. A lot of people want a fantastic body, and they put all of this emphasis on exercise and running and swimming and jogging and Pilates and yoga. However, if there's anything I've learnt about the body and what it looks like, it's that it's eighty percent what you put in your mouth and twenty percent exercise.

When I want to change my body, I don't reach out to exercise. I used to, but that's not what I do anymore. Now I reach out for cereal, avocado, sourdough, some lean meat, and substances that don't contain high levels of carbohydrates and fat. I do that for a couple of days or up to a week, to just reset myself.

This activates a trigger that gets me back on track. Nowadays, my weight parameters are anywhere from seventy-seven kilos up to eighty-three kilos, so I have about a five-to-six kilo buffer zone.

Any time I step on scales and see I'm beyond my parameters, I get back on track with my eating plan, which as I said is probably once every two years. Now when I travel I find it does have an impact, because I do love eating when I'm travelling. It just comes down to a basic wanting to try everything.

So for me it's that FOMO. You know, fear of missing out, and so when I travel I do have to find strategies, so believe it or not I'll travel with a box of cereal, because I've found that any time I want to reset, if I can just get my breakfast under control, then everything else falls in line. If I eat that cereal with some cold filtered water, it resets everything. I began to understand it serves as a trigger. So, the lesson is that getting one element under control will permeate the rest.

### Did you have cravings, and how did you mentally overcome them?

I think cravings are funny. A lot people try and use willpower when they're attempting to lose weight, and willpower is definitely a powerful resource, but I think what I've learnt over the years is that if I'm using willpower, I'm burning through a lot of blood glucose that I could be using for other activities.

As an example, if there's a Mars Bar in my fridge, and all day long I keep telling myself I'm not going to eat it, all of that mental energy I'm exerting could be used on something way more meaningful in my life. You may not want to hear this, but for me if there's a Mars Bar in the fridge, I've learnt just to eat it if I feel like eating it, because it's going to take me three hours of willpower not to, and I would rather use that time somewhere else.

Rather than having this thing called willpower, I've learned to adopt what a dear friend of mine, Dr John Demartini, calls *freedwill*. You know, not using willpower but freeing the will to go and do what's meaningful. What I've found is that you only have cravings when you're not doing meaningful work. If you want to avoid cravings and get your weight back on track, I can't offer any help, but I can say it's probably time you dedicated your life to some important purpose, otherwise you'll need to use willpower to overcome them.

It's been said that an idle mind is the devil's playground. Not that I believe in the devil, but I think it's fascinating, and the concept is quite true. Like when I'm busy creating a presentation or on stage presenting or on the telephone helping people transform their lives, I don't have time to think about eating a Mars Bar, because my mind is so active doing what I love that the thoughts that generate cravings have no space to exist.

I present two-hundred days a year all around Australia. During that time I eat just one small sushi meal, and that's it. Most people say if you want to lose weight you have to eat regular meals, and some say you need six meals a day to keep your metabolism firing. But I realised that if you're doing what you love, become immersed in it and listen to your body, you just don't get hungry anymore. One of my greatest lessons is to only eat when I'm hungry, eat more of what makes me feel light and less of what makes me feel heavy. It's not a tricky concept.

Whenever you feel hungry, drink a glass of water first and wait ten minutes. If you're still hungry, drink another glass and wait five minutes. If you're still hungry, then eat something. If what you eat makes you feel light, then eat a bit more of it. If it made you feel heavy and lethargic, then eat a bit less. This simple plan is the strategy of naturally thin people.

But thanks to marketing and a whole bunch of big business, people are convinced they must have breakfast, so the cereal companies can get their money. You must have lunch, so that cafes can make money, and you must have dinner, so supermarkets can make their money. It's important to stop and take a moment to consider who's telling you this information.

When you were a baby, you only ate when you were hungry, and when you were no longer hungry you stopped eating. No one taught you this behaviour, you just did it naturally.

But as you got older your parents said you had to finish everything on your plate, and you needed to eat at certain times. At school a bell goes off at one o'clock, and you have to sit down and consume a sandwich. It's just the most bizarre programming, and by the time you leave school you have this belief that you must eat at these specific times, and if you don't, then you don't feel normal. The mindset people need to have is to give themselves permission to choose their own eating journey. Just because someone next door has six meals a day, doesn't mean you're meant to.

There's an ancient shamanic principle that states the measure of truth is effectiveness, so what I always try to figure out is what's most effective for the individual. As you're going along your weight loss journey, it's critically important that you focus on, examine and hone that which is most effective to you at any given time, because it's how you get to know yourself at the deepest level.

One of the core principles I have to get across regarding core mindset shifts, is to eat when you're hungry and not just because the clock says it's time to eat. Too many people get this wrong, and I think that has an impact on their ability to experience the weight loss they're looking for.

In summary, I would say to forget about willpower. I'd rather eat a packet of Tim Tams than think about them all day in the cupboard, because it expends too much mental energy I could use to help change lives or write some training programs. It's counterintuitive, but you're much better off using all of that blood glucose to create something meaningful and make a difference in the world, as opposed to burning through all of that fuel just to not eat a Mars Bar.

**What mindset do you believe you need to be able to create weight loss success?**

I think it comes down to removing value conflicts. In our programs we teach a lot about this concept called shadow values, which is what clinical psychology would call secondary gain. With every action, there's a feeling that comes with it. Every minute of every day is filled with an action. For instance, right now I'm being interviewed and giving answers.

When the interview is finished, I could take the action of going for a walk and then for a ride, and later go to sleep, which is also an action. Even if you're just sitting on the couch doing nothing, that's an action. But every one of these actions has a secondary benefit in the form of a feeling, so shadow values are a culmination of feelings that people get from any activity.

I've done about two-thousand hours of research into this shadow value idea and tested it on hundreds of clients. After asking a series of questions I received a variety of answers, but I determined what the top seven were. The actions people take generally gives them one of these feelings:

1.  Attention

2.  Authority

3.  Belonging

4.  Control

5.  Rebelliousness

6.  Superiority

7.  Validation

What I've found is that if you're overeating, have an exceptionally heavy body or are embarrassed as a result of the way you look, you're getting something out of it.

Now, people say, "Well, Ben, I'm not getting anything out of it. I hate myself. I'm disgusted with the way I look", but the fact is they are.

People gain the weight, because when they had their body the way they liked it, quite often a trauma occurred. It may have been sexual abuse or a negative, violent experience, and when the trauma occurred, they stored in their memory the weight they were when it happened. Then they make sure they never go back to that weight again.

The brain's kind of a funny thing. It stores information. When a traumatic event occurs that shocks the system, to ensure it doesn't occur again the brain makes sure you don't replicate any of the elements of the equation. For instance, if you were riding a horse, then you stay away from horses. If you were in a certain location, you don't go back there. And if you were at a certain weight when this trauma occurred, you're never going to be that weight again.

When a trauma occurs, the body memorises the weight you were at the time and either makes you gain or lose significant amounts of weight as a protective mechanism. Quite often I've found with the people I've worked with, and quite a number of them are women, that unfortunately they've gained the weight because they no longer want a specific type of attention. This allows them to have a different outlook on how it all takes place. They will pad their body, because they still get the attention they crave at a deep, deep level, but it's negative attention where people insult them. It feels safer than if someone found them attractive and might come over and start talking to them.

Understanding shadow values is critically important in understanding how it affects your life. I once worked with a married man in a fifteen-year relationship. He was going to the gym and trimming down. When he got to a certain body fat percentage, he ended up cheating on his wife, and his relationship broke down. He also lost a large chunk of his money, so ever since then he's gained all of this weight.

Every time he'd try and lose weight, he'd get to within five kilos of where he was when he cheated on his wife, and then he'd gain all of it back again. His nervous system kicked in and told him that if he achieved it, he couldn't trust himself to control his sexual desires. He was a typical yo-yo dieter.

But understand this is all unconscious. Once this gentleman realised what was happening, we mapped his weight gain and loss, and he was honest enough with me to admit exactly what he weighed when he cheated on his wife. Then we were able to move forward.

**Why do you think it's important for people to have a great mindset regarding weight loss success?**

Everything you're driven to do comes from your mind. You can have a burning desire in your heart to want to change, but the mind is going to have to take care of the function and the voluntary actions that allow you to achieve your goals.

Mindset is everything. One of the simplest actions you can take to where you feel you're deserving of having the body you want is to understand your life is a manifestation of what you believe you deserve.

There's a big difference between desiring and feeling deserving. Everybody desires a fit, trim, healthy body, but deep, deep, down because of secrets and shames and guilt, they don't feel they're deserving of it, and so this permeates every area of life. But if health is the way you choose to sabotage yourself, then you have to get on track with deserving it. In life, the level at which you feel you deserve something, determines how much you will tolerate in any specific area.

I'll give you an example. If I don't believe I deserve to have a nice meal, then if I go to a restaurant and the chef cooks the meal inappropriately, my level of deservedness determines whether or not I complain about the meal or tolerate it. Now, if I believe I deserve the best food ever, that I work hard for my money, and I have no shame or guilt about the money I've earned, then I will politely send it back and ask for it to be re-cooked, because I deserve the best.

It's the same with your body. If you believe you deserve a great body, when it isn't looking the way you want it to, then you won't tolerate it, and you will complain. You'll politely explain to your body that this is not the way you want it to look. So when you look at a person's body, understand that this is what they believe they deserve, because it's what they're tolerating.

People need to change their mindset, because until they change the reference point as to what they'll tolerate, they will never fully change their body. One of the simplest actions I get clients to do is write out two-hundred reasons why they deserve a healthy, fit and trim body.

That is the absolute minimum starting point, and they need to read that list regularly. The next thing I would suggest is then linking it up to their shadow values.

As part of my chapter I'm giving away an audio program called "Shadow Values". It's going to help you get clarity on exactly what it is that's holding you back by doing some list writing around your shadow values. You can access it now at www.authenticeducation.com.au/shadow.

As I said earlier, I talk to a lot of ladies who don't like favourable attention, so a list I would get them to write is how trimming down their body and creating the physique they desire would give them more favourable or safe attention. This quite often allows them to get clarity on what they're doing moving forward.

The second list I get people to write is about how their healthy body would give more of the feeling they desire. For example, if they like to eat anything they want because it gives them a sense of control, then the question might be, *How will trimming down my body give me even greater levels of control?* Mindset will assist them in taking the voluntary action, because a region of the forebrain, called the telencephalon, is about voluntary motor control and coordination of outgoing movement. Until you get to the highest region of the mind, you're really taking involuntary action. In fact, up until that point you're just reacting to life.

If you don't have your mindset in order, you won't be able to reach the part of your brain that's responsible for voluntary body functions. And if you don't have voluntary control of your muscle movements, good luck trying to eat or drink healthy foods when you're hungry.

Unconsciously reacting to life is the number one reason your body looks the way it does. An event triggers you emotionally, so you eat without any thought process. Mindset is the quintessential element of weight loss. In fact, it's the quintessential element of anything you do from enlightenment all the way through doing inspiring work, and everything in between. It's your mindset that will give you voluntary control of your physical body, which can then perform the action that delivers the results.

We say in our company that life rewards action, so any result you desire, whether it has to do with weight loss, finances, career, business, family, friends or relationships, it requires action, and that action must be voluntary in nature, not reactionary, because those responses only get you what you've received in the past.

### How do you start your day?

Einstein pointed out the true sign of intelligence is imagination, not knowledge, and I'm a big fan of imagination and using it as much as possible. Before I go to sleep and when I get up in the morning, I spend a couple of moments with my eyes closed imagining the way I want my day to go.

The midbrain integrates both internal and external visual stimulation and allows you to experience and activate reward centres and experience and activate emotions and feelings inside the body. That's where the internal maps are stored that dictate what you do. What I've discovered after the psychological studies I've done is that your brain finds it virtually impossible to tell the difference between what's imagined and what's real. When I worked this out I realised I could literally shape my day and my world by just taking a few moments in the morning and evening to imagine my outcome.

I'm a big fan of meditation as well, and I believe that five to twenty minutes of good meditation in the morning is always going to put you in a great position to have more emotional control, which has a lot to do with your ability to maintain the exact physique you're looking for. Warren Buffet said that if you can't control your emotions, good luck trying to control your money, and if you can't manage your emotions, you'll never be able to manage your money. I think the same goes for your weight. You know if you can't manage your emotions, you'll never be able to manage your weight.

So in the morning when I first wake up, I lie in bed with my eyes closed and imagine my events full of people, my daughter's health, my wife's health, my family having a great life, my business growing and travelling. I imagine everything I love in my life exactly the way I want it. Then I do some basic gentle awareness of the breath from five to twenty minutes. It's a simple and easy way to start my day.

**What activities do you participate in that you never would have dreamed about doing as the previous you?**

One is going to pool parties. I know it sounds funny, but when I was struggling with my weight I would get invited to parties all of the time. When summer would come around, I'd start to get nervous. I'd covertly find out if there was going to be a spa bath or a swimming pool at the party, because my biggest fear was that halfway through, everyone would get their swimmers on, rip their shirts off and jump in the pool. So if there was any chance of that happening, I wouldn't go. I didn't want to run the risk of having to take my shirt off.

The beach was okay, because not everybody goes in the water, and someone had to look after the belongings, so I'd always volunteer for that job. But when you're at someone's house, it's different. Here I was this big, chubby kid sitting on the side of the pool while everyone else was swimming, and I figured I must look like a complete idiot. So if I got invited to a pool party, I'd suddenly have to go to help my brother out that weekend.

It impacted my freedom and my ability to do what I loved in life. And if I ever did jump in the pool, I would swim all day long and turn into a prune waiting until everybody had either gone home or gone inside, before I'd quickly get out. I never wanted anyone to see me climbing out of the pool.

I can go to pool parties now, and I never would have dreamed of it before.

**Is food or exercise the main contributing factor, and what food or exercises did you start out with?**

The answer would be food all the way. In my mind it's eighty percent food and twenty percent exercise. To be honest, I don't do any form of traditional exercise at all. Zero. I mean, I don't go to a gym, I don't ride a bike, and I don't jog. But I do speak for a living, so I stand throughout the day and walk up and down the stage. I've definitely found that when you're doing what you love and you're inspired by what you love, you do burn calories in the process.

I wouldn't suggest that people not exercise. I think it's important they do. My life is so busy, I exercise by walking and talking, and I certainly exercise by hanging out with my daughter and playing in the playpen with her. But for me it's all food. You are what you eat. My brother has a simple philosophy. He says, "Ben, if you eat for two people, you're going to look like two people." There are so many individuals out there complaining about their weight, but I watch what they eat and notice they're eating enough for two people.

I can appreciate there are those with physiological disorders, such as having their gall bladder removed or other parts of their body that assist in the processing of fats that have been affected by a disease. But a majority of people just don't realise how much they're eating.

### What's the biggest mistake people make when it comes to weight loss?

I think the biggest mistake people make, hands down, is that they try and remove items as opposed to replacing them. There's a functionality in the mind that says nothing is ever missing. Time is always full with something called space, and space is always full with something called time. There's no such thing as a void. Everything is always full, and your mind understands this. So if you say to your mind, "Hey, mind, I want to remove chocolate cake", then your mind says, "Ah, you can't do that, because there's nothing that's ever missing. If you try and remove chocolate cake and don't put anything else in its place, I'll bring it straight back."

I would advise people to learn the art of replacement. All change only goes through two distinctive steps:

Step one: Reduce your reaction

Step two: Replace your response

You probably played sport when you were in school but don't do it now, so you need to look at why you quit sport or how you went from a sport player to a non-sport player. For instance, if you played basketball in the afternoon when you got the desire to play, you reacted by picking up a basketball and shooting some hoops. Then later on in life when you got the internal desire to play basketball, you reduced your reaction and didn't pick up a basketball. Instead, you replaced this response with picking up the T.V remote. Voila, you're no longer a basketball player, and you've changed.

When you reduce your reaction but replace your response, change becomes easy. Before getting their weight loss under control, people make a list of what they're not going to do anymore, but my advice is to split that page into two columns. On one side write down what you're not going to eat, and on the other side write down what you're going to replace it with.

So when you get a craving for a Mars Bar, know exactly what you're meant to eat instead. For instance, you know that any time you feel like eating one, that actually means it's time to eat a carrot. Or every time you want to drink a high-carb beer, it's time to grab water. Or when you feel like overeating, it's time to take five deep breaths. You have to know what triggers what. I mean, in my own world I have a whole series of these, which I keep in my telephone. I call it my ROAR (Results Orientated Action Replacement), which is basically actions I replace to get the result I desire.

For example, thanks to Mark Zuckerberg, I have an internal craving to check Facebook daily. I don't want to keep doing it, but I also want to use the craving, because billions of dollars of marketing have gone into making sure I have it. So any time I feel the desire to look at Facebook

I call up a family member instead. This means for me, Facebook equals family time. Let's say I'm sitting at home and want to look at Facebook. Instead, I'll go and play with my daughter or talk to my wife. If I'm walking around the street and want to look at Facebook, I'll call up a family member or a friend.

Your ROARs have to do the same. The craving is always replaced and never removed. When you have a sheet like the one I've included below, which shows you a bit of a breakdown of the ROAR, you can determine what you need to stop doing to get the body you want and what you're going to start doing to replace it. Or what you're going to do less of and what you're going to do more of to replace it.

# ROAR

| What action do you need to stop doing? | What action do you need to start doing? |
|---|---|
| | Your Goal: |
| What action do you need to do less of? | What action do you need to do more of? |

For instance, you might decide to watch less television and do more walking. Or stop eating Tim Tams and start eating celery sticks. Then all of a sudden the brain understands what's going on. You're not missing television, because you've started walking instead. You're not missing Tim Tams, because you have celery sticks instead. The brain doesn't care, as long as it knows it's full. But any time you tell the brain that something has been removed, the brain will crave it until it gets the item back, and this is truly what craving is.

### If you had to start over again, what would you do differently?

I personally wouldn't change anything in my life for any reason, but if I was given the opportunity to start over again and I could take one idea back with me, it would be to have the power to appreciate all of my traumas, trials and tribulations.

I always tell people there's no such thing as a negative experience, just undiscovered value. Now I'm not a big fan of positive or negative thinking or any of those buzz words. I just think it's a good idea to appreciate life fully and completely. What I do know is that people can dig for diamonds in their life, so I'd like the ability to go back and discover all of the value it has. Like, if I got fired from my job, I would try to figure out what I could learn from that experience that I could use in the future. Or if I got abused as a kid, I could wonder what it taught me.

I would love it if I could do it all again with the knowledge and ability to instantly appreciate everything that happened in my life that gives me my wisdom, because it would allow me to learn and evolve significantly faster. Obviously you can't go back, but I think appreciating your life is critical, especially if you want to lose weight. You need to have that vibration of appreciation.

### What are your tips to having great control over your life?

I think to have great control over your life you need a fundamental understanding of shadow values and the importance of having a really strong *why* or purpose in life. It's about having a clear idea of the vision of what your life looks like. A lot of people remain stuck trying to make decisions, which are formed predominantly through emotion.

People wind up gaining weight thanks to not being able to control their emotions, and a lot of emotions are thanks to an inability to make decisions. So the best way to have control of your life is every single day to visualise the life you want exactly the way you want it. That way when it comes to day-to-day decision making, you have an internal future self with whom you can base your decisions.

If every morning when I get up I visualise myself standing on stage speaking to people, then throughout the day if I have to make a decision about something, I only have one question: does this decision get me closer or farther away from that image of me speaking on stage? If it gets me closer, then I say yes, and if it gets me farther, I say no. But just being able to make decisions more rapidly gives you great control of your emotions, and control of your emotions gives you control of your life. If you have control of your emotions, then you're able to lose the weight.

So I'd say it's critical to have a vision of your future self that's inspiring and lights you up. That really connects with you at a heart level. If you visualise and imagine it daily, you'll easily be able to recognize in every situation what brings you closer to that vision and what will distance you from it.

### What techniques do you use to achieve your goals?

I'm a big fan of falling in love with the process. For instance, you don't see Roger Federer out on the tennis court in the middle of his training session saying, "Geez, I can't wait for this training session to finish, so I can stop practicing this forehand. All I want to do is win a tennis championship." People at the top of their game don't think like that. These professional athletes, you can't get them off of the tennis court.

They play all day, every day, regardless of what they're doing. Falling in love with the process is critical to goal achievement.

People tend to fall in love with the outcome. You may imagine six-pack abs, but if you don't love sit-ups, really love them, then good luck getting that six pack. If you don't love the challenge of pushing yourself to do one more sit-up when every muscle in your body is burning, then you're going to find it difficult to achieve. I love creating presentations and designing coaching sessions. I love tweaking and modifying strategies for transformations, I love doing research and presenting and I love doing interviews like this. So for me, goal achievement comes down, first and foremost, to loving the process. If you don't fall in love with the process you'll be really hard pushed to get the result.

I would also say it's understanding the power of reverse engineering. I like to get my goal into the smallest bite-sized chunks possible. Kathy Sierra, a computer programmer, did a talk in Silicon Valley in 2012. She spoke about something called deliberate practice, which is where you break down a goal you want into such small steps, that each step only requires a maximum of three sessions to get it to world-class level.

So if I wanted to achieve the goal of, say, violin playing, I would break it down into the smallest possible tasks. First I'd practice picking up the bow. If I picked up the bow for three solid hours, eventually I would be able to do it at world-class level. Next I would try picking up the violin, and I would do that for three sessions until I could pick up the violin to world-class level. Then I would place the bow on just on one string and take it off repeatedly, until I was at world-class level. This is a deliberate practice anyone can use to achieve anything. They need to be willing to break the goals down small enough, where it only takes three sessions to get it to world-class level, but most people sabotage their goals by making their actions too big.

Like, let's say you want to lose twenty-five kilos. That action is too big. A better action is to go to Rebel Sport and buy a pair of sneakers. That's a tangible action. Then the next action could be to put your sneakers on and walk around your house for a week, which gets you used to wearing them. The next step is to walk to your letterbox twice every Monday and after that to do a lap of your block.

Now if you persist with this style of small actions, within six months you'll be jogging around the entire suburb. But if you start with the idea of losing twenty-five kilos, you'll feel overwhelmed and sabotage yourself. In the end, it's breaking down the goal into small pieces and deliberately practicing each one. Here are the steps:

1.  Fall in love with the process.

2.  Break it down into smaller chunk sizes.

3.  Look for habits, not goals.

A habit-oriented mindset says that if you want to write a book, forget about writing a book. Just form the habit of writing four-hundred words a day. Even if you wrote a hundred words a day every day of your life, every couple of years a book would fall out of you whether you liked it or not. Habits allow you to complete a series of actions on a regular basis that delivers your goals, whether you like them or not.

I think it was Aristotle who said that we are what we repeatedly do. I believe success is a habit, so look at what you're doing habitually, day in, day out.

**Is there a significant quote or saying you live by?**

There is one quote I tend to live by. Art Linkletter said "Things turn out best for the people who make the best out of the way things turn out". The way I understand this quote is that it's the ability to say wherever I am in life right now, I'm going to make the best of it. If I weigh two-hundred kilos, I'm going to make the best of it. If I'm unemployed, I'm going to make the best of it. If I'm bankrupt five times, I'm going to make the best of it. If my heart has been smashed into a million pieces, I'm going to make the best of it. Everything really does turn out best for the people who make the best out of the way things turn out. I actually live by that quote.

To discover more about how Ben can help you *Elevate Your Health*, visit

www.elevate-books.com/health

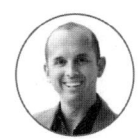

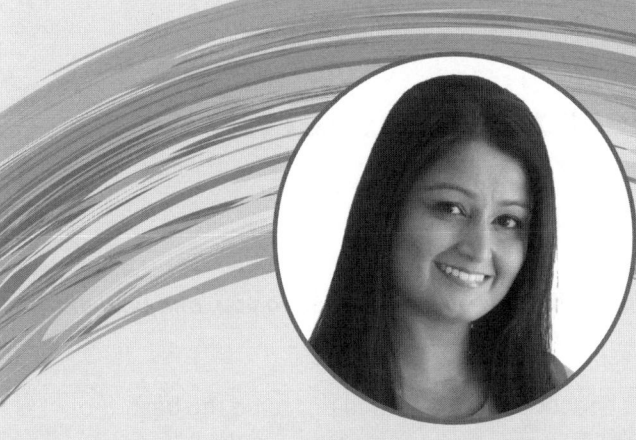

# Ameeta Gangaram ND

## Endless-Energy

Ameeta is a qualified naturopath, herbalist and nutritionist with over ten years of experience. She specialises in adrenal fatigue recovery and assists her clients to create vitality and enjoy more energy naturally.

Ameeta's passion for helping people with adrenal fatigue is due to firsthand experience, as well as taking part in practitioner training to better support her clients throughout each stage of their recovery.

Ameeta runs a successful clinic, Zest Health Centre, in Brisbane, Australia, where she delivers her Endless-Energy Program, as well as personally tailored programs designed to reset the body on the pathway to health that leaves clients feeling energised, calm and in control again.

Ameeta is a presenter and author, and in her free time loves dabbling in art and photography.

# Ameeta Gangaram ND

## Endless-Energy

**What's the worst thing that has ever happened to you, and how did you overcome it?**

The worst thing that happened to me turned out to be the best, too!

If you were with me in 2007, you would have witnessed me make the bold decision to quit my job as a naturopathic assistant in a pharmacy and open up my own business. I'd become disillusioned with the way businesses were being run and the nature of focussing only on increasing sales, without any attention being paid to the actual needs of the customer.

The over-prescribing by doctors and pharmacists went against my personal ethics. There was no concern for interactions, diet, lifestyle and the actual cause of their dis-ease, which I define as when your body is so out of balance, it's unable to repair itself due to lack of nutrition, poor lifestyle choices and an increased amount of stress. It seemed there was always a pill that could fix it all. I didn't want to be a part of this process. I was determined to show people that running a business in the health industry could be done with the clients' best interests at heart.

And so my organic health food store and naturopathic clinic, Organic Matters, was born. I created a space that was safe and filled with whole foods, natural goodness and nutritional supplements of the highest quality, all ethically formulated. Customers came in knowing they were getting honest advice every time. My education and can-do attitude meant that my customers got the help they needed for themselves and their loved ones.

The problem arose when I realised I was giving so much of myself to everyone around me it started to affect my own health. I had run the business full time, working sixty-plus hours a week for nearly four years. My amazing mother resigned from her job in order to assist me with my business. She was my pillar of strength. Still, all of the administrative responsibilities and behind the scenes running of the business sat solely with me. This meant I couldn't take a holiday. I had to be at work six days a week, and along the way I sacrificed my friendships and all of the activities I loved like exercising, art and travel.

After nearly five years of being the heart and soul of the business, I started to fall apart. My energy plummeted, and I felt exhausted and drained all of the time. I became overly emotional and would go from happy to sad to angry in a matter of minutes. My sleep, which I'd always loved, became erratic, and I felt un-rested when I awakened. The worst part for me as a naturopath was that my diet fell to pieces. I started relying on chocolate and sugar to give me some kind of a boost in the afternoon, and I hated myself for it. I also cried in my car a lot. My weight increased seemingly overnight. Looking back, I realise it was so hard for me to understand what was happening and stop myself from doing it.

This pattern lasted several months, until one day when a customer walked in and without me even saying a word, said she would come back another day when I was in a better mood. Wow! I was so shocked and appalled with myself, because it meant what I was feeling on the inside had seeped out and was on display to the world. Something needed to change, and it had to happen fast. This is when it first hit home that I was suffering from adrenal fatigue. I realised the way I was feeling was not normal and that it was due to me pushing myself too much. I had forgotten to find a balance between work and my personal life and didn't have any good stress management tools in place.

The thing is, it suddenly became the best thing that could have happened to me. I made the choice to let go of my business. As much as I loved my store, it wasn't serving me well. The concept of

Zest Health Centre emerged at this stage. My dreams developed into having a clinic that focussed on helping to prevent people from going down the same path I had.

Two weeks after finishing up with Organic Matters, I found the ideal clinic setting in Mitchelton, which is in Brisbane, Queensland. This clinic was opened so I could provide the long-term support I knew people needed and present my clients with the steps to achieving optimal health. My programs within the clinic are designed to guide and teach people every step of the way.

### If could speak to your younger self, what advice would you give?

If I had the opportunity to speak to my younger self, there's so much I would love to say. The key topics would have to be these:

1.  Believe in yourself.

    You're amazing and have a wealth of knowledge to share with this world. Your compassionate nature and ability to give of yourself are traits this world needs. Your message is worth sharing, no matter how big or small, and your voice can help others with their healing journey. This will create a ripple effect for them to help their fellow human beings.

2.  Take care of you.

    Your health and wellbeing should always come first. If you're not well or strong, then you won't be able to care for those around you. It means listening to your body. Don't overdo it. Find the time and activities that help you to release stress and find your endless energy.

3.  Strive to be better.

    Never let complacency take over space in your heart and mind. Obstacles in life are an opportunity to experience something new.

Embrace them, and you will be amazed by the positive changes that come about.

### What do you think you've been put on the planet to do?

I feel my purpose in this world is to help as many people as I can to better understand their health and the reasons they feel ill, overwhelmed and stressed. During my time practicing as a naturopath and herbalist for over a decade, I've seen a trend of people working longer hours and placing too many demands on themselves. My role as an educator is to show people how they reached their place of ill-health and dis-ease and show them the steps to reverse and heal their bodies.

You may not realise your work environment, as well as your diet, lack of exercise and stress management, are all part of why you feel exhausted, overwhelmed and anxious a lot of the time. The burden on your body, hormones, and more specifically your adrenal glands, becomes overwhelming. The adrenal glands are really quite incredible in that as a species, we depend on them as our primary survival organs. They're responsible for helping to cope with stress. Everyone has these two walnut-sized glands that are situated on top of the kidneys. They play a vital role in the body's endocrine (hormonal) system.

The adrenal glands control the fight-or-flight mechanism. For instance, when you're in danger. It can even happen when you think the boss is going to fire you, you're worried over money problems, have anxiety over the health and wellbeing of your kids, or are nervous about the welfare of your marriage and other relationships. There are nearly unlimited amount of worries you carry around at one time or another, and the adrenal glands mobilize all of your resources to fight or get away from that danger. They're small, yet so powerful. They're like the key to a treasure chest. They can unlock wonders for you if you just know how and what they need, and I'm about to give you the key to unlocking your endless energy.

Historically, the immediate dangers humans have faced were typically short-lived. For example, running from a sabre-toothed tiger. When this system gets activated, a hormone called cortisol is pumped out from the adrenal glands, which makes the thought process more sharp, gives energy and mobilizes blood sugar to fuel the muscles. Breathing becomes faster, and the heart rate goes up to prepare for high-energy action. Once safely out of harm's way, the chemical process is resolved, and everything goes back to normal. Another hormone, insulin, pumps out and mops that extra mobilized blood sugar back into the cells. As a result, breathing and heart rate go back to normal, and all is once again well in your world.

You've probably seen vivid examples of the fight-or-flight mechanism on the Nature Channel. There are gazelles around a watering hole. They're calmly drinking water, when along comes a lion. Now the chase is on, and there's all kinds of action. Once the lion catches a weak, sick or elderly gazelle, what do the others do? Go right back to calmly drinking at the watering hole again, as if nothing happened. This is a clear representation of what the nervous systems should be doing.

 My goal is to help people recover from adrenal fatigue, no matter what the stage, as well as prevent it from occurring in the first place. There are simple methods you can implement to start feeling energised, healthy and happy again. It's the reason I created my Endless-Energy Program, available in-clinic or via Skype/online. More details can be found by visiting the link at the end of this chapter.

### What is adrenal fatigue?

Adrenal fatigue is a condition caused by some form of stress. It can be physical, emotional, mental, environmental, infectious or psychological. It can even be a combination of these.

The adrenal glands act as shock absorbers for the body. They help you bounce back from life's many stressors. When you're under too much, or unrelenting stress, eventually the adrenals get tired of working overtime, which leads to adrenal fatigue. This is when you start to experience symptoms such as tiredness, allergies, insomnia, irritability, anxiety, depression, recurring infections, arthritis, and difficulty concentrating and retaining information, as well as struggling to lose weight.

Instead of me randomly listing more symptoms, I'd like to tell you about one of my clients. Leanne is in her late forties. Her energy levels started to deteriorate after she picked up a bad bout of the influenza virus. She became so tired, that at work she noticed herself dozing off in front of the computer. This was even occurring in the morning, when she usually would wake at five am for her daily yoga practice and meditation that she loves. Being a yoga teacher, she knows the importance of exercise, but her body wouldn't allow even this level of activity, due to her complete lack of energy.

She'd also been trying to lose weight for years, but it wouldn't shift. She was so rushed during work hours that she hardly had time to eat or would eat while on the run. Her days were full, as she's a manager of a retirement village. She would become frustrated and moody with her husband on a daily basis, and she knew this wasn't normal. It all became too much for her to cope with, so she decided to take two weeks off work, just to relax and get some rest in the hope that it would be enough to restore her energy levels and have her feeling calmer and in control again. When this didn't work, she called me.

When she came in and told me about how she couldn't even get out of bed in the morning, that she'd become moody and her sleep had deteriorated to the point where she was waking every hour, I knew that it all stemmed from her adrenal glands.

I explained that it was because of the major stresses and pressures of her job and also that the virus she picked up really was the tipping point for her energy and vitality being affected so negatively. She listened and decided to take action.

After a month on the Endless-Energy program, she reported that she was waking up every morning at half past five and doing a one-hour yoga session, followed by thirty minutes of meditation. One month prior, she hadn't thought it was possible.

### What are the symptoms of adrenal fatigue?

There are three stages to adrenal fatigue. In each stage, the symptoms differ.

1.  Alarm Stage

    This is the beginning of it all, when you're burning the candle at both ends. The alarm stage is when you feel *wired but tired*. You have enough energy throughout the day, but when you sit down in the evening you crash and fall asleep in front of the TV. You might also then get into bed but lay awake for ages, because your mind won't switch off.

2.  Resistance Stage

    This stage develops when you haven't listened to your body and keep working long hours, so you're not resting, and your adrenals can't keep up with the demands you place on them. Your adrenals' cortisol production decreases due to exhaustion setting in. You start to feel anxious, exhausted from the time you wake up, irritable with everyone and get colds or chest infections on a regular basis.

3.  Exhaustion or Burnout Stage

    As the name suggests, this is the stage when you've depleted all of the stores of nutrients and hormones. Your adrenal glands just can't keep up, and the fine balance within the body breaks down or topples out of control. All of the symptoms of the first two stages can be present but are much worse and are plaguing you all of the time. You can't get out of bed, which results in not being unable to hold down a job. You become emotionally fragile because of fluctuations in blood pressure and blood sugar levels. You suffer from depression and can feel that life is just too much to cope with.

Below is a summary of the common symptoms you might experience in each of the stages. It's important to note you may have some of these or a different set of symptoms. This is because every person is unique, and so is the way the body presents adrenal fatigue and other conditions indicating ill-health.

| ALARM | RESISTANCE | EXHAUSTION/ BURNOUT |
|---|---|---|
| • Tired in the evenings<br>• Falling asleep in front of the TV<br>• Insomnia – struggle to fall asleep when in bed<br>• Coffee/caffeine is required for energy, especially around 2-4pm | • Recurring infections<br>• PMS symptoms<br>• Insomnia – frequent waking at night<br>• Anxiety<br>• Irritability and moodiness<br>• Naps are needed | • Blood pressure changes<br>• Extreme exhaustion to the point where time off work is needed or doing your job is impossible<br>• Dizziness<br>• Anxiety<br>• Depression<br>• Mental fogginess |

**How do you find out if you have adrenal fatigue?**

There are two ways. The first is to answer an in-depth series of questions. These are designed to give your naturopath or health care practitioner detailed insight of your health, past and present. I've listed the first ten questions I like to start with.

Exercise: Answer the ten questions now with a *yes* or *no* to find out if guidance from a qualified naturopath or health care practitioner might be of benefit to you.*

1. Do you wake up feeling exhausted?

2. Do you skip breakfast?

3. Does your head feel foggy, and do you struggle to focus and remember things?

4. Have you noticed you're becoming more sensitive to certain foods?

5. Do you suffer with hay fever, sinus problems or headaches?

6. Have you had a major traumatic event in your life, such as a divorce, loss of a loved one, loss of a job, marital problems or a car accident?

7. Do you crave salty or sweet foods, especially in the afternoon between 2-4pm?

8. Do you need a coffee in the afternoon as a pick-me-up?

9. Have you noticed that your sex drive has decreased?

10. Is it harder for you to handle stress?

*The results from these questions are informational only and not intended for diagnostic purposes.*

The second way to find out if you have adrenal fatigue is the Rolls Royce of testing. It's a twelve-hour Salivary Adrenocortex Stress Profile. This is the test I use for all of my clients on the Endless-Energy Program. This hormone, or stress test, serves as a critical tool for uncovering biochemical imbalances that underlie anxiety, depression, chronic fatigue syndrome, obesity, blood sugar irregularities, and a host of other health issues that may be affecting your day-to-day life. Salivary cortisol testing is the most accurate and powerful non-invasive hormone test that evaluates the levels of the two most important stress hormones:

cortisol and dehydroepiandrosterone (DHEA). This test will help you understand in what stage of adrenal fatigue you are currently and the steps that need to be taken in order to rebalance your body.

***Do you have an approach to treating adrenal fatigue?***

I've had huge success with my clients that have completed my Endless-Energy Program. This five-step program provides you with all the support you need:

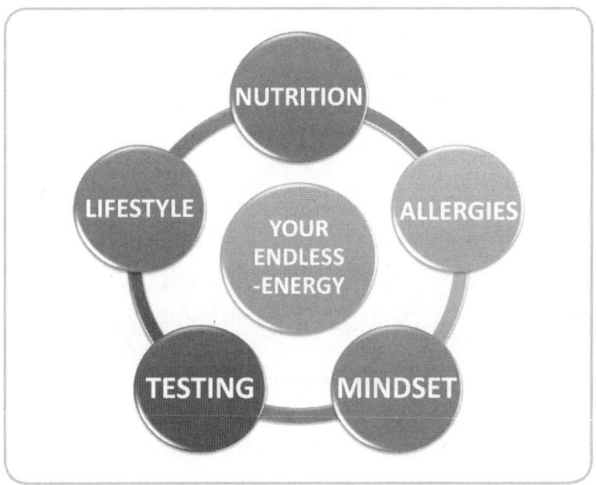

1. Gravitate to good nutrition

2. Alleviate allergic reactions

3. Embody a healthy mindset

4. Test your adrenal gland function

5. Strive for a balanced lifestyle

During the program, you're provided with all of the tools you will need. The reason for these steps is to heal your body on a physical, emotional, mental and physiological level. At the same time you're developing new and healthy habits to stand you in good stead for the future. Healing the body allows for balance to be re-established and your energy and vitality to return. You're given all of the support and nutritional supplements you require. Your diet and lifestyle are all thoroughly assessed, and a plan of action is then developed just for you. All of my consultations can be done at my clinic, Zest Health Centre, located in Brisbane and Sydney, or via Skype or online. For more information, contact me at info@zesthealthcentre.com.au

I also go into a lot of detail about each of these steps in the workshops I run, called, "Create Endless-Energy: *The fastest way to experience more vitality in your life right now.*" These are run regularly. Come to one and find out more valuable information that can help you feel healthier and happier.

I've found that if you don't focus on each of these five steps, over time you will end up feeling the same or worse. When you follow this program, you know you're going to feel like a new you!

### What is your most inspiring client story?

That would have to be Anne*. She was falling apart when she came to see me. She'd been suffering with constant hay fever and was relying on antihistamines daily for over a year. She was waking up exhausted every morning when she'd run out the door with no breakfast and work long hours after a forty-five minute drive to work. She was also a fulltime mother and wife, while doing post-grad studies at the same time. Anne would fall asleep on the couch after work, with no energy to make dinner for her husband and son. This meant relying on take-away meals several times a week. She started having chocolate in the afternoon, just to get through. At night when she got into bed, no matter how tired she was, she couldn't switch off her brain and would lie awake for hours. This resulted in her feeling even worse, and her relationship with her husband started to suffer. She just wasn't coping.

So what I did first was start her on my Endless-Energy Program. It taught her how to listen to her body, rest, repair the nutritional deficiencies and use relaxation techniques to mentally release her blocks. It turned everything around for her. She felt motivated again and ate well throughout the day. She felt so great, in fact, that it rubbed off on her husband and son, who both gave up chocolate and junk food as well.

This newfound energy allowed her to travel overseas for a holiday. While there, she had boundless energy, no hay fever and enjoyed the company of her family.

Now you understand that working towards optimal health benefits every aspect of your life, and positively impacts the lives of those you love.

*Name changed for confidentiality purposes*

**What's the biggest mistake people make when they're exhausted and suffering with adrenal fatigue?**

I think the biggest mistake people make is to think it's perfectly normal to feel tired every morning and to struggle throughout the day. They think everybody else feels this way. The problem this thought pattern causes is that people leave it until they can't get out of bed or some major health disaster occurs, before they seek attention. It's definitely not normal to feel like this. You should wake up refreshed and happy. Your mood should be stable, and you should be able to sleep well every night, without disruption. Coffee shouldn't be your best friend. Instead, it should be water.

My wish for everyone who may possibly be suffering with adrenal fatigue is to listen to your body. When it says *I'm tired* or you start feeling run down, lethargic and have recurring infections, do something about it. Call me or a naturopath and address it now. Your healing time will be so much faster, and your body will love you for it.

### What's the best way for someone to transform their energy levels?

Action is the key to transformation. I always tell clients at my events and in my clinic, "You've taken the first step today by being here." And so have you by reading this chapter and being open to healing yourself. That deserves a pat on the back. Go ahead and do that right now.

The second step is to find out in what stage of fatigue you are. Like I mentioned earlier, there are three stages: alarm, resistance and the burnout or exhaustion phase. In order to find out, come in and take the twelve-hour Salivary Adrenocortex Stress Profile. Once you have the results, a plan will follow as to what your body requires in the form of supplements, lifestyle changes and relaxation techniques.

Think **S.L.E.E.P.**

1.  **S**uccumb to sleep. Try to get between seven and eight hours a night. This will allow your body to heal and feel energised. Rest on the weekends if you need it.

2.  **L**imit your intake of sugar and caffeine. Both will make you feel even more tired over time.

3.  **E**liminate foods you're sensitive or allergic to.

4.  **E**xercise gently. Small amounts of the right exercise can be beneficial, but if you're in the exhaustion phase, then it's vital to limit exercise initially, in order to recover.

5.  **P**rovide protein to your body. Think of protein as the bricks to build your house (body).

### Why is health so important?

Looking after your health can provide you with a valuable lesson: *self-love, awareness and taking action will result in an abundance of vitality and happiness.* This has the benefit of improving every other aspect of your life, including your mindset, career success and relationships. Start your day with the right frame of mind, and see how that plays out through your day.

This is crucial to how I feel and what I can accomplish. I certainly love my morning routine and have seen it greatly improve my productivity. It's a process I learnt when I did one of my courses with Benjamin J Harvey. My version of the routine goes like this:

I wake up at six am, lie in bed with my eyes closed and visualise every hour of my day, exactly how it's going to play out. For instance, what I want it to feel and look like and what I want to achieve. Upon opening my eyes I verbalise five things I'm grateful for in my life. Gratitude brings on a sense of peace and positivity. You truly have so much to be grateful for in your life, and when you verbalise it or write it down, it sinks into your core, and you carry this feeling throughout the day.

Akshay Dubey says, *"Healing doesn't mean the damage never existed. It means the damage no longer controls our lives."*

I'd like to share five tips to improve your health:

1.  **Water is essential.**

    Aim for a minimum of eight glasses of pure, filtered water.

2.  **Have breakfast every morning.**

    A simple boiled egg, oats or even baked beans are a great start to your day. Skipping breakfast usually means you wind up eating too much food at your next meal, because you're starving by then. You also eat the wrong types of food. The key to breakfast choices are that they should be high in protein, fibre and micro-nutrients. That sugary cereal is just not going to cut it, I'm afraid.

3. **Swap your coffee with green or dandelion tea.**

I know you love your coffee, because it gives you a pick-me-up. In reality, coffee makes your situation worse. It's depleting your body of essential B-vitamins and has also been shown to recreate stress conditions, due to cortisol being released from your adrenal glands. This means you're left feeling more stressed and agitated than before.

4. **Include protein-rich foods in each meal or snack.**

Protein helps to regulate your appetite and keeps you fuller longer.

5. **Cut down on starchy carbohydrates.**

These have a high glycaemic index (GI) and offer you less valuable nutrition. If anything, they leave you feeling more lethargic after eating them.

These are just some of the tips included in my workshop, "Create Endless-Energy: *The fastest way to experience more vitality in your life right now*" and my Endless-Energy Program. If you'd like to learn more, please visit the link below.

 To discover more about how Ameeta can help you *Elevate Your Health*, visit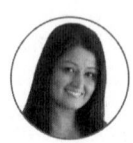

www.elevate-books.com/health

# Shivi Chhabra

## Harmoniously Balanced Women

Shivi Chhabra is an author and holistic health coach.

In her quest to find answers for her own complications related to polycystic ovary syndrome, Shivi has spent nearly ten years researching women's health issues. In the end, she was able to cure her PCOS naturally and gain an understanding as to what true health really means.

Shivi's love of natural health solutions and inspiring woman to live a better life helped her transform her own life. She now devotes her time and energy to helping women deal with hormonal issues and ignite in them a lifelong desire to take care of their body by looking at every aspect of their health.

Shivi assists women across the globe to achieve harmony and have total balance of mind, body and environment. Through her unique, proven techniques, she helps women who are ready to live the fulfilling life they truly deserve.

# Shivi Chhabra

## Harmoniously Balanced Women

### Getting closer to your feminine side

Before you start, sit calmly, close your eyes and imagine a slightly positive shift happening in your mindset and health. Take a few deep breaths, and open your eyes. Now imagine this feeling whenever you have an aha moment while reading this chapter.

***When and why did you first become interested in curing hormonal imbalances?***

Many women struggle with hormonal issues and issues around their womb. Despite advancements in medicine, this is one area that remains unknown regarding women's health.

I began my journey of curing PCOS, which stands for polycystic ovarian syndrome, when I was sixteen. It's the most common endocrine disorder in women and was first recognized in 1935 by Doctors Stein and Leventhal, but until now there's been no cure for this condition or a complete understanding of its cause.

Western medication does everything possible to mask the symptoms by using synthetic hormones to hide the symptoms that can be seen with the naked eye. They harm your body by slowly teaching it to forget how to naturally manage your hormones, and in addition impact your stress levels and emotional health.

After realizing the long-term impact of these medications on my health and years of exploitation through medication, I was ready to take my health into my own hands. When I began my journey there was no way of understanding this specific area of women's health due to lack of

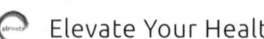

information, as well and the unwillingness of doctors to explain what happens inside the patient's body.

I finally had enough and wondered how hard it could get. Every expert advises you to change your lifestyle, such as eating clean and exercising every day for thirty minutes. No one told me what eating clean and exercising really meant. Thus began my journey of self-discovery.

Not long after I was done researching, I tried quite a few methods and still saw my health going in a downward spiral, so I decided to become a personal trainer. What could be better than knowing the answers firsthand like an expert?

But personal training didn't help, as the fitness industry lacked the knowledge and consideration regarding a woman's body being different from a man's, and thus their fitness levels are different as well. Excessive exercising without enough knowledge of how a woman's body works, particularly in respect to her hormones, can easily reverse the impact of the hard work expended.

So, my journey continued. I looked beyond diet and exercise and invested my energy into educating myself about the female body and the intricacies of hormones. My focus on the emotional aspect of my health led me to what was missing, which was my understanding and acceptance of myself and my femininity.

### So, what's femininity?

It doesn't mean a feminist agenda of fighting for equal rights with men. Don't get me wrong. I totally support and appreciate all women have been able to achieve in terms of equal rights, and I'm blessed to have been born in this era of freedom.

I'm just a little more concerned if fighting for equality has led women in the direction of being and having what men have. What if we're not supposed to? What if you have something better, but you decided to overlook it in this competition? It's purely human nature to ask and fight for what's being denied, and sometimes it's good to stop and ask why.

***What are these rights of femininity, and why are they so important for women?***

For eons, women have been channelled and taught how to be in a patriarchal society. Even though times have changed, women still find a need to constantly remind men they're equal and can't be suppressed.

The good news is that you're not equal, superior or inferior to men. You're some lucky souls who got blessed with a female body and were given some amazing gifts to have this human experience in a way no other living creature can.

Some of the beautiful rights/characteristics/gifts/powers of being a woman are:

- celebrating your intuition and sixth sense

- having the entire human experience of life and death every menstruation cycle and an opportunity to learn something new from it every time

- acknowledging your powers and finding ways to use them to care, nurture, share and love

- accepting the sheer power and magic you have to create life within you

- having forces that activate your body's inherent capacity to heal itself

- understanding your connection to nature, such as how it feeds your spirit

- understanding, knowing and influencing your innate capabilities and leading your own tribe

- reaping the benefits of being a woman and experiencing the world in a way no man is capable of

It's important to understand and apply these correctly, because it brings women closer to who they are and aligns them to themselves. They'll look at some of the more important roles in their life, which may feel forced and a burden, as more beneficial. Women will see the world from a different angle of feeling well deserved and lucky to be one.

### How do women find these feminine characteristics within themselves if they don't think they possess them?

Acknowledging some of these characteristics could be a daunting process, especially if the opposite has become so ingrained in your personality. But the truth is that everyone has these characteristics, and the sooner they're acknowledged, the easier it will be to live life to its potential.

When you've been told all of your life that you're the inferior sex, less capable, more dependent, delicate and fragile, it's hard to acknowledge these powers. For your outer world to change, for people to become more accepting of you with your new abilities, it's important to change on the inside.

Using the table below, you could identify these characteristics in order to realize you not only possess them, you've always had them.

| Quality/characteristic or power | What it means | Instances that prove I possess these qualities. |
|---|---|---|
| Intuition or sixth sense | Using your intuition and giving it credibility. Letting it flow and help you when you need it. | When has my intuition helped me? These are examples of when I decided to trust it, and the results were astonishing. |
| A new life lesson in every cycle | Every cycle lets you find out what's working for you and what's not and gives you an opportunity to grow a little bit every time. | What changed in my last cycle? Was there something substantial I realised about life? What did I change that actually worked? |
| Power and magic: creating life | Celebrating your capacity to create miracles inside or outside of yourself in any area of your life. | How many small or big projects have I created and completed? How are they serving each other? |
| Forces that activate the body's inherent capacity to heal itself | Believing in yourself and your body's healing capabilities. | When has my health gotten better when the situation seemed hopeless? How was I surprised by the outcome? |
| Connection to nature, how it feeds the spirit | Women get their energy by being more connected with nature. You believe nature and humans are one. You serve each other to coexist. | When did I feel more energetic and connected to myself and something higher while being in nature? How do I feel about animals? |

Elevate Your Health

| Quality/characteristic or power | What it means | Instances that prove I possess these qualities. |
|---|---|---|
| Care, nurture, share and love | By sharing, caring, loving and nurturing, you feed on oxytocin (love hormones). | How many times have I shown care and love towards someone or something? How many times did I find an opportunity to nurture something or somebody? |
| Innate capabilities of knowing, influencing and leading | You have this ability of knowing. You sense the need and at times take a higher road for the greater good of your loved ones. You find ways to encourage or instigate them to grow. | What are the instances when I've encouraged or even instigated helping someone I love to take a leap of faith and follow their heart? |

## What relation does being more of a woman have with curing hormonal issues?

If you look at the past month of your life, how many times did you feel you should or shouldn't be doing something because you're a woman? All of these thoughts and feelings reinforce the idea, consciously or subconsciously, that being a woman is a bad thing.

Most women link these negative emotions to a natural behaviour of their body. For example, when you have your cycle, it's uncomfortable, painful and annoying. Your hormones work synchronously, creating a melody that either sounds beautiful or discordant. These hormones are responsible for a web of communication that triggers responses that feed all other vital organ in your body, and the cycle continues. This is true for menstrual cycles. It's a perfect example of the delicate communicating web of hormones. You can read more on this subject at: www.studiohealthevolution.com.au

This delicate web is susceptible to changes in your mind, body and environment, and hence brings up the concept of holistic health. Your thoughts, perceptions, feelings and emotions contribute many folds to your body's reaction to external factors. The image below shows how this delicate web works.

The pituitary gland that sits at the base of the brain is important in controlling growth, development and functioning of other endocrine glands, which secrete various hormones throughout the body. A part of the peripheral nervous system, the autonomic nervous system, acts largely unconsciously and regulates bodily functions like heart rate digestion, respiration and hormonal responses.

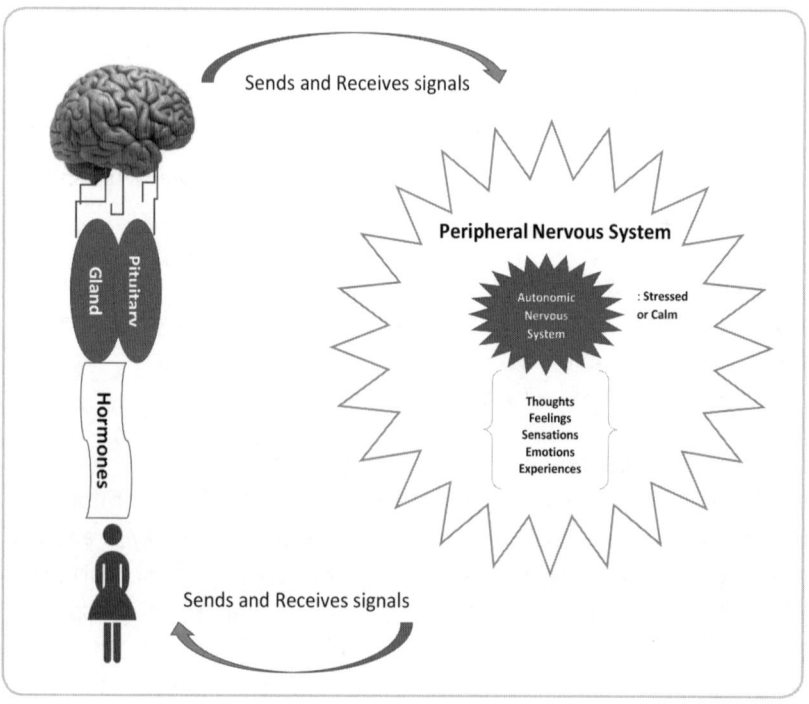

Your brain works in mysterious ways. Your subconscious mind picks up all signals, and your body's autonomous nervous system responds by either staying in balance or activating the flight or fight response to protect you from a threat or stress, both perceived and actual.

The surprising part is that your brain doesn't distinguish between an actual or perceived stress. This pressure in the life of a woman misaligned with her feminine self could be generated from many situations and circumstances in her day-to-day life. Any event that makes her feel helpless can be perceived as a threat by the brain. As long as the brain stays in the fight-or flight-state, the body won't work in balance. The autonomic nervous system is responsible for working nearly all of the body's systems, and the endocrine system is one of them. The longer you stay in this state, the more harmful it is for your body. Over the course of time, you create habits that feed onto this state of fight or flight as your body gets used to it.

The good news is there are ways to break through these patterns, and that's through mindfulness. Being aware of these thoughts and patterns could easily help you identify what meaning you're giving to certain experiences in your life and how they're keeping you off balance and impacting your hormonal health.

**What's mindfulness, and why is it so important? Are there quick ways to be mindful right away?**

Mindfulness means being aware or watchful. It keeps you in the present moment and frees you from the time dimension of past and future where you wander most of the time.

In Buddhist practice, mindfulness has four foundations. I will cover three of them, as they're related directly to health. Mindfulness is one of the ways of lightening your feminine powers by activating your senses and making you aware of your hidden thoughts and patterns that constantly keep you in a state of fight or flight.

Your consciousness is in the balance of mindfulness of body, as well as sensations and feelings (emotions). This balance maintains a rhythm that's responsible for all of your life experiences: pain, pleasure, happiness, sadness and dullness, anxiousness, fear, love, affection and hatred. When you become aware of your feelings and sensations in your conscious mind, you become more balanced.

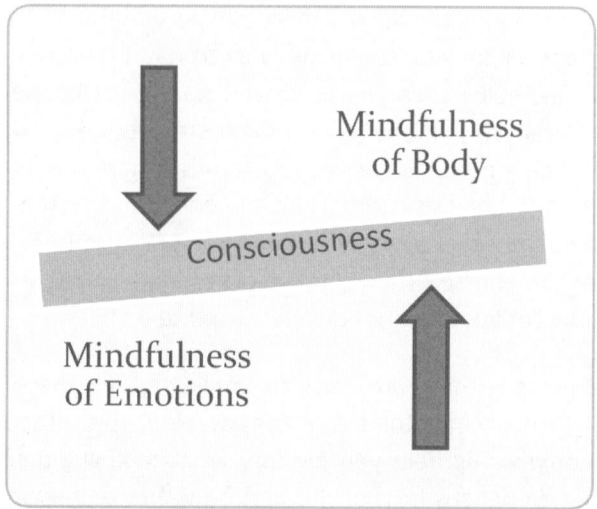

### Mindfulness of the body

Mindfulness of the body is observing your body, in whatever shape of form, as a medium to view and experience the world and not the reason to live in it. The world seems to revolve so much around how you look that it's become a reason to live and is responsible for your happiness and sadness.

Women should look pretty to attract men, while the definition of pretty keeps changing. Nowadays, the definition of beauty is more in the form of an unachievable and generalised definition of a good body image. It seems like a way of distracting women and keeping them from realising their powers.

There are three core pillars needed to be mindful of your body

1.  Integrating mind and body

    Integrate your mind and body, so the focus remains aligned. This could be achieved through your day-to-day activities and meditation. A simple activity where you're focused on a task, such as gardening, is a perfect example.

2.  Being in the now

    Your mind loves the time dimension you've taught it through the ages. If your thoughts are mostly concentrated on the past or future, it takes the focus away from the now and keeps you from experiencing certain signals your body is sending. Staying in the now means being more in tune with your body.

3.  Focus

    Focus is concentrating your energy and directing your attention in a particular direction. When you focus your attention and energy on your body, you listen to it more. It tells you pretty much everything you need to know at any a given time. Are you hungry? Full? Enjoying you food? Just compensating your feelings and emotion with other physical behaviours and habits? Focus on breathing and being meditative.

While being mindful of the body, it's important to remember that as soon as you see a negative pattern of behaviour, don't react or get judgmental. Acknowledge it, stay focused and try to find out a way to satisfy your needs by asking yourself these questions.

1.  What do I really need right now?

2.  What can I do to give myself what I need?

Once you receive your answers, act on them immediately.

**Mindfulness of sensation and feelings**

Women are remarkably efficient at suppressing their feeling and emotions for the greater good and the roles they play in society. These feelings are eventually ignored, because they've been told to, or it's become a habit as they move through life just believing what others tell them. They carry these negative energy fields while adding to them.

The end result is health deterioration. The most commonly ignored and denied emotions are anger and anxiousness. These are the signals the body gives to bring attention to certain aspects of your life. You class every sensations and feeling as good, bad or neutral, and the body reacts by having cravings or aversions. For you to be mindful of these feelings and sensation, you must:

- identify and observe the feeling and sensation by knowing where it is in your body and then acknowledge it while showing no emotion or judgment and not categorising it

- let it pass through you smoothly, like a flowing river

- identify if it's a good emotion and enjoy it, but don't get attached to it

- record it in order to find more patterns over time

The best ways to identify feelings and sensations is by being still and meditating.

**Mindfulness of mind**

Consciousness is emotive, rather than intellectual. It represents mindset or state of mind. It's responsible for creating experiences in thoughts, speech and actions. When your mind and heart are disconnected, it's hard to get hold of your thoughts, which are induced by actions and feelings. Perform the following steps to be more mindful of your mind. Use meditative focus to understand if you're focused, distracted, agitated, calm or stressed.

1.  Observe your thoughts. Watch them like a spectator

2.  Acknowledge them and show no emotions or judgements. Don't react

3.  Let them pass through you like a flowing river

4.  Don't judge or categorize them as good or bad

5.  Once you've finished observing, if you've noticed a pattern during meditation, ask yourself these questions:

    ▸ What are my hidden fears and anxieties, and how are they related to my thoughts?

    ▸ Is there any other way I can address them, so they don't occupy my mind and impact its state?

### What contribution does food and exercise have in balancing hormones?

Food and exercise play an important role in health, which I consider an ongoing process that works like sand through an hourglass. When the sand is gone, you're ready to topple and start again. The top half of this hourglass is filled with knowledge you must gain to improve your health, and the bottom half is nutrition and exercise, which is the base that supports this model.

Nutrition and exercise are essential steps in improving a woman's health, but they're not the only ones. You must have heard this saying:

*You are what you eat.*

In my opinion, this is not entirely true. You're also what you think, treat and believe yourself to be.

Real food nurtures you, gives you energy and makes you capable of achieving goals. Its role is to ensure you get everything your body needs to make you capable of enjoying your life to the fullest.

In my last ten years of research I understood one concept, and that is until your mind and heart are aligned, you'll see no results. This is true with food and exercise. If your heart and mind aren't aligned with what you're putting yourself through, you get no results.

Not long ago I developed a bad relationship with food. It originated from all of the diets I tried in my pursuit of curing my PCOS, which was also the reason for my frustration and bad health. Even though I never went on a yo-yo cycle, at one point in time I was sugar free, dairy free, wheat free, gluten free, meat free, processed free and was on a low carb diet at the same time. If you're curious to know what worked, the answer is none of them. I added in all of the *free* over the course of four years while trying for something that might work. The short-term results gave me some confidence, and I never wanted to take the *free* out. Yet I wasn't happy. It frustrated me and made me wonder what I was missing.

Soon I realized that whatever shape, size or weight I was, either small or large, I never felt happy with myself. I wasn't aligned with my feminine self, and that led to constant tiffs between my conscious and subconscious self. Whichever won at a point in time decided my actions and feelings. This realization was quite profound and made me question a lot of other decisions I'd made in my life. It was like a breath of fresh air.

Here are a few simple questions I asked myself to attain the body type I wanted.

1. What do I *really* want from my body, and why is that important to me?

2. Is it what I want or something I've been influenced to want?

3. If my body is bigger or smaller, fatter or slimmer, stronger or weaker, then what am I comparing it to and why?

4. Do I know what it will cost me, such as money, time or other sacrifices? Am I willing to pay the price?

5. Would it make me happy? If yes, for how long? Could I sustain my results and happiness?

The answers resulted in making good decisions about my health.

These questions are relevant to exercise as well. Women are the most exploited gender in terms of consumerism. A single idea or expression could be moulded in several ways to feed insecurities, like for instance a model on the cover of *Vogue* with an unachievable body. You get influenced by stereotypes and this incessant need to fit into one of these boxes.

It's quite amazing to see what lengths women will go to in order to achieve these results. On the plus side, women are getting stronger and more equipped with skills to manage their own health. Also, they're getting fitter and more conscious of what they're eating and how they're taking care of themselves.

But they must also consider why they want to achieve these goals. For many, strength is a way to showcase they're as strong as men or to demonstrate rebelliousness towards suppression. At times it's purely a form of protection. By answering the questions, you would know if you're in sync with your heart and mind. There's no right or wrong answer, only truth. If there are reasons you're moving further away from your femininity, they need to be addressed. Being mindful would help you identify the core reasons.

Exercise has shown to improve hormone health in woman, but this exercise may not be for a beach body. Instead it's to improve your daily life. Exercise is a way to get you closer to yourself by taking care of this beautiful gift that lets you have the most wonderful experiences. It improves breathing, and this might be the only time you concentrate on your breath the whole day. Listen to your heart pound in your chest and be present. Go beyond your cycle of pain. It could be the way to rejuvenate yourself and concentrate on you rather than everyone else around you. This new way of looking at exercise made me like it more, have more fun with it, and understand it didn't have to be painful.

### How does someone know if they're in sync with their feminine side?

You'll know you're in sync with your feminine side when:

- you're okay being vulnerable and are happy taking chances

- you have newfound love for your lady parts and show gratitude for them being there in their perfect shape and form

- you have a new desire to dress up, love yourself and feel good

- the incessant need to be in control of your life fades away, and you're happy to share responsibilities and be a team player again

- you help other woman grow without having the need to be superior

- you don't judge women who are closer to their feminine side and are happy to learn from them

- you feel more free and yet in control of your life

- you acknowledge your powers and find ways to put them into action

- your body seems to cooperate with you, and there's newfound love of taking care of yourself

- the feeling of being suppressed seems to fade away, and there's a new perspective on being a female

- your hormones are back to normal, and there are signs of ovulation and clearing skin

- you have more energy and confidence

- your self-esteem grows

- you see the issues related to differences in the male and female sex as less inciting

- you like your own company more, so "I'm bored" seems like a silly statement

**What do you think inspires people, and do you think it's important to have goals?**

Having a purpose and a vision is so important. I feel women have immense power to create magic in their family, career or business. Women often get restless when they're purposeless. Give them a project, and the situation turns around.

A channelled energy is much more useful with a sense of purpose. By setting up small, achievable goals that ultimately feed your life purpose, you'll realise your powers.

Download your free audio on how to set your health goals at www. studiohealthevolution.com.au/health-goals

**What's the most common fear woman have towards changing their lives and achieving their goals?**

I once asked a client what her deepest fear was when it came to changing her life and claiming her power. She said not being able to do it. When asked if her feelings would be the same if she had all of the help, time required, and resources she needed to achieve her goals, she replied that it wasn't how much effort she had to put into it but what she'd have to change around her to do it. She figured she wouldn't be able to give her friends and family the attention they deserved, so they wouldn't like the changes and start treating her differently. Then she'd wind up doing everything herself and be left alone.

I've been astonished that the number one deepest, darkest fear women have is being left alone. So many women feel that having improved health, a better life and standing up for themselves would change the perspective their friends and family have towards them. This is the simplest yet most dangerous example of giving power away and going leaps and bounds to please someone, even if it doesn't serve them. Family, friends and partners must support you in your journey.

Women must preserve their powers and channel them in a more productive way that serves them, so they take care of themselves first. The right to acknowledge their powers, execute them and ensure they're seen and respected by others, is one of the most important actions to get closer to their femininity. Women have been taught that showing love means pleasing and putting others first and themselves last. This teaches the people in their life to see them as less important.

***What's the best way women can help themselves overcome this fear?***

When you make a decision, the universe aligns itself to help you achieve your goals. What you need are SMART goals. Here are some general rules for obtaining them.

**S**pecific

**M**easurable

**A**ccording To You

**R**elevant To You

**T**ime Free

Yes, I said time free. People tend to put themselves under a lot of pressure thanks to businesses, schools, religious ideologies and society in general that teach if they fail or make a mistake, they must be punished and beat themselves up. This is done by going even harder and failing even more miserably.

You deny your needs, curse, mistreat yourself, increase negative talk and at times physically hurt yourself. You treat yourself like your body is a different person that's not letting you be happy. *If only I could have dropped five more kilos. If only my arms were slimmer, If only I'd made a little more on that deal. If only...I would have been happier.* When your happiness lies on the other side of success, and success seems to change dimensions, then you'll never be happy. This unhappiness is reflected in many areas of your life. A failure in one area is in fact a failure in all, isn't it? You carry on this baggage of guilt and shame everywhere. You can't even hide it, because it's you.

It's within your power to change this whole cycle by having SMART goals you build every day and improving your self-esteem. This will take you closer to your life purpose, so you get closer to your femininity and learn to love yourself. It's much easier said than done, and it may seem like it takes forever, but you need to:

- be comfortable in your skin

- understand why you're here

- understand why it's required to look inside first

- understand other people's opinions just don't matter

Having goals gives you purpose and a sense of achievement. It gives you a reason to take back your power preserve it and protect it.

Download your free audio on how to set your health goals at www. studiohealthevolution.com.au/health-goals

### *What do you do when your decisions go wrong?*

1. Get back up

2. Dust off

3. Pat myself on the back for the efforts I made

4. Learn from my mistakes

5. Move on

I ensure the whole process takes only a few seconds. Life is too short to be wasted on regrets and remorse.

**If you were speaking to your younger self, what advice would you give?**

▶ Embrace your femininity and refuse to listen to people who tell you to walk, speak or treat others a certain way.

▶ Don't try and match your peers.

▶ Don't be embarrassed when you hit puberty and refuse to be body shamed.

▶ Be your own best friend.

▶ You must follow your way. It will work. It's all going to be okay.

▶ At some point in life you will fight for the right *to be*. Not doing it now means you'll do it later, or if not then life is going to show you how someone else's way isn't working. It just depends how long you're willing to wait.

▶ Your intuition guides you, your will empowers you, your perception creates you and your imagination liberates you.

▶ There are powers that protect you, energies that connect you and forces that heal you.

▶ Make the decision to listen, know yourself, love yourself and acknowledge your power, now and forever.

▶ Remember who you are and what you're capable of, which is being free to live your life in your own way.

**Are there any daily rituals to keep someone on track?**

Journaling and mediation with mindfulness are the best ways to get back on track with yourself and your health.

Your menstrual cycle can be divided into four phases, representing your spirit and temperament. If you've reached menopause, then map these days to the lunar cycle, where day one is the new moon. A lot of women have already started to implement this structure in different ways. I derived my inspiration from *humoral theory* but have adopted it to match some of my own needs.

| Season | Temperament characteristics | Day in the cycle | Questions to ask |
|--------|------------------------------|------------------|------------------|
| winter | calm, thoughtful, patient, peaceful | 1-7 | What did I learn in my last cycle? |
| spring | courageous, hopeful, playful, carefree | 8 – 14 | What new changes am I ready to implement in my life? |
| summer | ambitious, leader-like, restless, easily angered | 15 – 20 | What am I ready to reap in this cycle? |
| autumn | despondent, quiet, analytical, serious | 21 + | What am I ready to give up in this cycle? |

Keep a diary and answer these questions for each of the phases.

▶ How do I feel today?

▶ Is there something I need right now?

▶ Did my day give me an opportunity to fulfil my need?

▶ What activities are easier for me to do at this phase?

Pick a question relevant to your phase questions to ask from the last column of the above table.

Continuous use of this format to record your thoughts and feelings will give you a good picture of what works best for you in each of these phases and could be used to plan your cycles accordingly.

**How can someone bring loved ones onboard? Could they be of any help?**

Yes, having your partner by your side learning and growing along with you is beneficial. Bring them up to speed by looking at a few educational videos on the topic at www.studiohealthevolution.com.au.

In the end, it's your journey, but be cautious as to who you engage. It's about you connecting with yourself and listening to you. If there are people who want to be more right than you are and want to override your own influence on yourself, then I suggest you take a step back. As you gain power, your environment changes and people change. In the end, you need to have a strong connection with yourself. Either people will understand your journey by joining you or they will slowly move away. It's a two-way street.

**Do you have any last words of wisdom?**

The hardest thing I had to do in my life was to slow down, understand my needs, get more aware and match the pace of my world with my actions. But it's by far the best gift I've given to myself. Sometimes just standing still helps. It's your time to stand still. Take a moment to know yourself.

You can only go as far in your life as your understanding of yourself, so how far are you willing to go?

To discover more about how Shivi can help you *Elevate Your Health*, visit

www.elevate-books.com/health
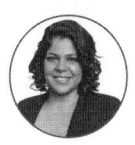

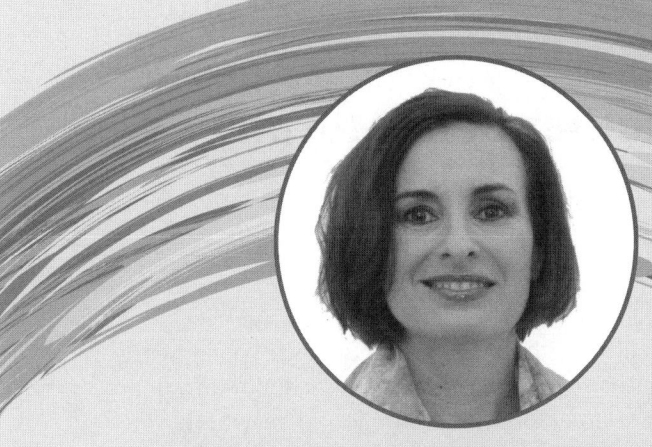

# Heather Belle Murphy

## Keeping A Breast

Heather Belle has been an environmentalist, naturopath, educator and speaker, acting locally and thinking globally, for over twenty-five years. When she was a child, she had a chronic illness that went undiagnosed, and as a result she suffered from anxiety and depression. Then as a teen she was sexually molested and developed an eating disorder.

Following a visit to a natural therapist, she became captivated with nutritional and quantum medicine, which combined with an innate desire to help others, has become her lifelong love and primary mission.

Since certifying as a naturopath from the prestigious Southern School of Natural Therapies in Melbourne, she has also added hypnotherapy, wellness and relationship coaching to her qualifications. Heather Belle also presents regularly to peers and various community groups, has volunteered with the long-term unemployed and focuses on women's health through Neuro-Emotional Trauma Release and as a Cancer Recovery Coach. Currently, she's working toward completing her first book, *The Truth About Men*.

# Heather Belle Murphy

## Keeping A Breast

> "You can search throughout the entire universe for someone who is more deserving of your love and affection than you are yourself, and that person is not to be found anywhere. You yourself, as much as anyone, deserve your love and affection."
>
> ~ *Siddhartha Gautama, The Buddha*

### What is your big WHY?

I doubt there has been a family in the Western world that hasn't suffered the loss of someone special to cancer. Some families even seem to be overrun with it.

My life has been touched by the loss of my maternal grandmother, Doris, due to breast cancer. I never got to meet her. I only have the photographic evidence of being cradled in the arms of a sweet, smiling woman who looks a lot like my own mum. What should have been a joyous time for my parents, with the imminent arrival of another child, was instead imbued with sadness and impending loss. Mum experienced her pregnancy with me knowing her own beloved mother had been given a near-future death sentence.

My parents, in particular Mum, then juggled two children and a difficult newborn baby, all while caring for an increasingly ill loved one and watching powerlessly while she simply wasted away. I was eighteen months old when she died.

Several years ago, Mum had a scare and underwent a procedure to remove malignancies from one of her breasts. As I haven't had children, I'm aware that statistically I have an increased risk of manifesting breast cancer. Bearing that in mind, just over a decade ago I experienced my own scare with a manually induced lymphatic problem that created several painful lumps in my left breast.

> "I have always believed, and I still believe, that whatever good or bad fortune may come our way we can always give it meaning and transform it into something of value."
> ~ Herman Hesse, Siddhartha

That incident prompted a shift for me. It was an awakening that brought me into the *now* and forced me to check in with myself. Where did I actually think I was going, and how would I get there?

At the time, and I readily admit this, I'd veered off my preferred life course. I'd become like so many women I meet almost daily. I was too busy and worked too hard, while putting aside more meaningful needs with an unrealistic schedule. I felt stressed and relied somewhat on emotional eating, including biscuits, cakes or chocolate to sweeten my life, and I enjoyed too much wine too frequently, which put on extra kilos of weight that I hated. Generally, I had a sound Business Plan but my personal Love-Life Plan had slipped with the demands of my business and a highly driven partner who was like a force of nature. I needed to look at the bigger picture, detoxify physically and allow for more *Me Time*.

### *What exactly is the problem with Cancer?*

"If you go to the doctor with a headache, and the doctor provides you with a prescription for aspirin and the headache goes away, does this mean you have an aspirin mineral deficiency?"

*~Dr Joel Robbins, Health Through Nutrition*

From a holistic viewpoint, the presence of cancer is not *the problem* as such. It's the symptom of a deeper underlying condition. Focussing on *fighting* cancer. including its removal, poisoning or suppression, and as so often happens, chasing it around other parts of the body to find and kill it, will sooner or later kill us.

In the first place, standard Western medical cancer treatment substantially increases physical trauma for an already ill person, drastically increasing stress and therefore, ironically and tragically, increasing the cancer risk. It also doesn't address the underlying cause for the presence of the disease at all.

To put it in perspective, in the 1950s the risk of cancer for people under the age of sixty five was approximately one in ten. Recently, the Australian Bureau of Statistics has reported it at one in two. That's in spite of the hundreds of millions of dollars spent on research.

In 2014, Cancer Australia expected one in eight Australian women to be diagnosed with breast cancer that year. And even though the five-year survival rate is expected to be eighty-nine percent, with credit given to earlier detection and improved treatment, it's still the second leading cause of cancer-related death, with the risk still rising. In my view, not nearly enough attention is placed on prevention. Recent statistics from an Ovarian Cancer Australia fact sheet reveal that in

2015, 1,480 Australian women were diagnosed, and 1,040 of them will die from the disease, with only a forty-three percent five-year survival rate.

So you have to wonder if Western medicine on the whole treats cancer by putting out the fire with gasoline. I would answer resoundingly, YES. This is in keeping with a report by the American Cancer Society, published December 2014, titled, "Secondary Cancer", which admitted the risk of the high recurrence of difficult-to-treat cancers after radiation and chemotherapy treatment.

There are many issues to be addressed.

Firstly, a much more proactive approach to the prevention of cancer is needed and much overdue. Well-documented risk factors for cancer aren't being addressed adequately by the medical profession or in society at large, for instance, dietary-related factors such as the obesity epidemic, diabetes and heart disease. At no other time have we ever been more overfed and inversely malnourished.

Secondly, Western cancer treatments aren't only immensely physically traumatic and quite toxic, they add significantly to emotional stress and the intrinsic stress of the situation. Stress being a direct causative agent in influencing the spread, or greater likelihood, of metastatic cancer has just begun to be more fully investigated.

According to a recent episode of ABC-TV's *Catalyst* program, one research team is estimating the risk of cancer increasing sixfold, with a direct stress correlation. The role of Beta-Blockers in reducing the physical effects of stress and increasing the longevity of breast and ovarian cancer sufferers has been documented since 2010.

Another offshoot is that some patients have been so damaged by aggressive treatment they become lifelong human guineapigs of immune-suppression and sometimes chemotherapy regimens. This is a very real problem, for example with the increased risk of suffering drug-induced leukaemia being well-documented.

Thirdly, in not addressing the primary inflammatory cause of cancer with obvious diet and lifestyle modification, secondary cancers are likely and will be less responsive to further chemotherapy, which has been documented by the American Cancer Society.

Over the last few decades I've spoken to many sufferers and families firsthand, and it's my opinion that most people are ill informed about their health. They're actively discouraged from taking a more proactive stance by the medical profession in relation to diet, exercise, lifestyle and stress management, which could obviously reduce the need for treatment and therefore the fallout from side-effects and recurrence.

That's not to say I would dissuade anyone from pursuing a conventional medical path they saw fit to follow. However, no one can deny that being better informed and taking greater responsibility for their health is likely to produce a much better outcome not only for the sufferer, but the family and community at large.

### But isn't cancer hereditary or genetically programmed?

No, I don't believe that's so. I think that idea is a misunderstanding of a bigger picture. While of course it's true that humans can carry genes for a particular genetic expression, they have a trigger or switch. Are you living or loving in such a way that will switch on that disease pattern?

Depending on the source, five to ten percent of women carry genetic mutations that supposedly increase their risk of breast cancer. Lately, there have been some well-known women opting for double mastectomies rather than risking the same fate as other family members. However, it's well documented that Japanese women experience minor incidences of breast cancer compared to Western women. Their traditional diet has been found to be cancer risk reducing, because it's rich in antioxidants and plant isoflavones.

Over a decade ago, I worked with a client whose mother had died from bowel cancer several years before, and she was worried she would suffer the same fate. I've no doubt she would have been right if she hadn't come in to see me for a complete health makeover. She was morbidly obese and chronically constipated. She was eliminating what she considered regularly but was actually once every four days! She was a busy working mum who spent over two hours a day commuting to work.

I first recommended a few colon cleansing appointments to aid her most major channel of elimination. Her colon must have been really backed up, so she was reabsorbing toxins back into her bloodstream that would normally have been eliminated. Plus she was at risk of a possibly life-endangering bowel perforation and blood poisoning. Yikes!

We made some simple dietary changes, such as reducing processed sugary snacks, increasing hydration, soft, soluble fibre, and most importantly, green veggies. She made time for a minimum twenty-minute walk daily and arose ten minutes early so she could relax on the toilet until she'd reconnected with her body's signal that it was time to evacuate.

Within a few months, she had transformed into a goddess! She looked like her younger sister. Her mottled, bloated look was replaced with a peaches-and-cream complexion, and she'd lost about twelve kilos simply due to eliminating waste as nature intended.

She quickly realised she was pushing herself in too many directions and began keeping an eye on commitments, followed shortly with the added benefits of greater productivity and peace of mind. Cyclically and hormonally she also felt much better, as her liver could now function properly. She was bright-eyed and bushy-tailed.

> "Your beliefs become your thoughts, your thoughts become your words, your words become your actions, your actions become your habits, your habits become your values, your values become your destiny."
> ~ *Mohandas K. Gandhi*

### What is cancer?

Simply put, cancer is a label given to the uncontrolled division of abnormal cells. First of all, for cancer cells to thrive, the healthy cellular environment must be absent. Secondly, the immune system is "asleep" and not performing its protective role, most likely due to cellular malnourishment and toxicity. Think of cancer cells thriving or not thriving in laboratory test tube conditions. The body is a chemical soup. For cancer cells to be generated and thrive, an unhealthy environment must maintain them.

The important question to ask is, "Why would this be?"

As a practitioner of holistic and preventative therapies, I don't treat anyone for cancer or disease. I work with people by following a holistic philosophy that the whole is greater than the sum of its parts. Another way of looking at it is that humans aren't simply a version of Dr Frankenstein's Monster, a conglomeration of parts animated by an external force. We have an innate vital force, or electromagnetic field, that in the case of imbalance and disease has been suppressed.

### Do we really have a vital force?

The answer is a resounding, YES! People are light energy-based spiritual beings having a human physical experience. Jedi Master Obi Wan Kenobi, wasn't kidding when he advised Luke Skywalker to "Feel the Force", in a classic tale signifying the archetypal hero's journey. As the regular person comes to know thyself and steps beyond the limitations of the everyday and embraces becoming *The One*, they take responsibility for their actions, beliefs and fate to the best of their ability.

What is The Force? It's the energy the universe is made of, including human beings. And while humans think they're made of solid matter, they are in fact a moving field of atoms vibrating at a rate dependent on their atomic makeup. What are atoms made of? Neutrons, electrons and positrons. What are neutrons made of? Smaller energy particles.

> "You are not a drop in the ocean, you are the ocean in a drop."
> ~ *Rumi, Thirteenth Century Persian Mystic and Poet*

### What difference can raising my vital force make in the role of disease?

Everything has a vibration or an electromagnetic field that can be measured, including the formation of all disease. Therefore, to be capable of producing cancerous cells, a body must be vibrating at that rate. As Bernard Jensen, the man recognised as the father of modern naturopathy and holistic medicine wrote, *We don't 'catch' cancer. We create it by the way we eat, breathe, think, drink and live.* He advocated tissue cleansing and nourishing whole foods, including the application of the seven doctors, which are sunshine, good food, pure air, clean water, exercise, healthy habits and mindset.

How does someone know if their vital force has decreased? Physically, it's easy to tell. There's a lack of energy, general good health and radiance. Common factors that will diminish your vital force include

- anxiety, depression, obsessions and long-term aggravated stress

- smoking, excess alcohol or drug abuse, including prescription medication

- little or no exercise or conscious stress management

- poor quality foods and a highly artificial diet

- not enough sleep on a regular basis and poor living habits

- unchecked morbid obesity and elevated blood sugar levels

- no healthy future outlook, including a life plan

Another factor that most people don't yet recognise as a significant problem is electromagnetic field radiation from devices that are increasingly everywhere.

People live beside antennas, sleep next to giant TVs, sit behind car batteries and even "fresh" food is surrounded in fridges by electrical fields and plastic. If smoking a packet of cigarettes daily has the equivalent radiation of a chest x-ray, imagine the effect of holding a lithium battery next to the brain for extended periods or the habit some women have adopted of keeping their phones in their bras.

### Can mindset really make a difference?

Again, a resounding, YES!

About thirty years ago, I first heard of affirmations and creative visualisation after reading Louise Hay's groundbreaking book, *You Can Heal Your Life*. About sixty years ago she was diagnosed with terminal cancer, and today she's a self-healed survivor who recovered using a combination of diet, lifestyle and changing her mindset. She's now eighty-nine years old and still works as a Light Healer and inspirational figure worldwide.

We're also incredibly lucky here in Australia to have the centre set up by long-term breast cancer survivor Olivia Newton John. She credits a big change in diet and lifestyle, including regular meditation, alongside modern medicine, with her healthy survival.

Although Traditional Chinese Medicine is thought to have originated over five thousand years ago, including linking emotions energetically to organ systems, the benefits of meditation have been largely discounted and overlooked. In spite of studies going back to the 1970s that began to prove physiological health benefits in regular meditators from lowering blood pressure, to reducing the levels of the stress hormone cortisol, to improvements in brain function. The link between meditation and its role in recovery from cancer has now been proven beyond a doubt.

In 2014, findings of a Canadian research team were written up in the *Cancer Journal*. They studied the effect of meditation on telomere support. Telomeres are like DNA tips on the end of chromosomes. As they degenerate, people age. They're the latest direct indicator of cellular aging. During a three-month study of patients undergoing Western breast cancer treatment, the telomeres of the control group shortened, while there was no change in the group of meditators.

This study has massive implications for not only prevention but the development of an integrated oncology approach. Perhaps this could also help to prevent chemotherapy-related toxicity, where the immune system is so aggravated it turns on itself and results in organ failure and death from a cytokine inflammatory storm. Cykotine are small, secreted proteins released by cells that have a specific effect on the interactions and communications between cells. A cykotine storm is a potentially fatal immune reaction consisting of a positive feedback loop between cytokines and white blood cells, with highly elevated levels of various cytokines.

Or if they're "lucky", a survivor will suffer lifelong debilitation.

Overall, the idea that emotions impact health and the development of disease is not new. Even the conservative USA Centers for Disease Control and Prevention (CDC) has stated that eighty-five percent of all diseases appear to have an emotional element, but the actual percentage is likely to be much higher.

Dr Bruce Lipton's *New Biology* is another school of scientific thought that adds to this way of thinking about disease, namely that emotions can trigger genes to either express health or disease.

Bear in mind that the health of the immune system is largely controlled not only by diet but by conscious and unconscious mindset. The role of the importance of mindset has been largely ignored by Western medicine. For example, the new psychologies of Neuro-Linguistic Programming and hypnosis have been studied and proven to bring about physiological changes, such as lowering blood pressure. I have the direct, regular experience of hypnotising clients out of decades-old habits such as smoking, in an hour. Just imagine the positive input it can have on the survival brain to switch from a fearful or pathologically functioning mindset to that of a healthy one, simply by changing the script.

### Why is love an answer to cancer?

Previously, I had a common female mindset that I was like a water well. I thought it was my role to give out love endlessly, like drawing water out of a well, even when I was low on resources, emotionally or physically. In those days, I had a lot of parasitic "friends".

I now know it's a common device women use to distract themselves from confronting issues of self-worth. It's a way of having unconscious needs met without having actual needs met. I over-functioned in my close relationships, appearing really competent, while feeling like a failure. It's a common, unconscious insecurity and control issue for women who "love too much".

Shortly after commencing practice as a naturopath, I saw a lady who had cancer of the spine and been given six months to live. Previously she'd had a double mastectomy and a few years later a full hysterectomy. Listening to her schedule made me exhausted. Where was the support in her life? It's unfortunate I didn't have the skills in psychological reversal that I have today. The idea that she was sacrificing herself by putting the perceived needs of her family entirely before her own was unfathomable to her.

It's amazing how many women confuse personal sacrifice to their families as a form of love. You can't give away what first you don't have. That attitude is nothing short of suicide-martyrdom. And yet, it's an uphill battle when women who seem to be doing it all and living as the Ultimate-Self-Sacrifice-Superwoman-Mother Martyr are upheld as pillars of society. I know it's confronting and shocking to realise that most often the loveliest and nicest women you'll meet would rather endure having parts of themselves removed, undergo awful drug regimes or indeed die mothering everyone else than begin to respect, honour and love themselves.

Tragically, it's normal for women and mothers undergoing a health crisis to distress themselves further by trying to keep up a brave appearance so the rest of the family isn't upset. I have no doubt that feeling unable to express authentic fear and grief contributes to terminal outcomes. That's where my immense life experience and having personally confronted death without fear, can be of real service to families undergoing an immensely challenging time.

A much healthier mindset for women is to see themselves as a fountain of love. Fountains self-water. This means women give to themselves first from the spring, and the lovely water splashes off, thus refreshing others. It's like the instructions parents receive on airline safety briefings that tell them to give themselves oxygen first before putting the mask on the child.

I'm sure that as my early childhood was greatly influenced by anxiety and insecurity, I unconsciously modelled myself on those patterns. That was my idea of normal. At the time, I assumed everyone felt immensely self-conscious, ashamed, guilty and responsible for situations that were wrong in the world. Those thoughts inversely kept the early developed survival part of my brain safe.

In pretty much the same way that I modelled myself on my mother and smoked for years, even though consciously I hated smoking, I couldn't stop until I'd worked out the unconscious need that was being met. A process of psychological reversal released the addiction. At the time, I blamed smoking as the problem, which was a form of suppression. Literally, a smokescreen for low self-esteem, anxiety and lack of healthy emotional processing or neuro-emotional detox.

Of course, those survival instincts are inbuilt to protect you, for example, when you sense some kind of danger. But at times they may keep you trapped in bad modelling or poor programming. People's lives today, here and now, are a direct representation of the programs and filters being run by their unconscious minds.

To put it in another more relatable way, your day-to-day wants are forebrain, conscious-mind driven. For instance: I want to lose ten kilos/I want to be rich/I want to marry a nice a person. The unconscious, survival-hindbrain-driven needs are what you actually create. *I want to lose ten kilos* comes from the conscious mind that includes willpower and being rational and analytical. *But I need to be overweight, because I believe/perceive that my family/ friends/ teacher didn't love me or I don't love me*, stems from the unconscious mind that includes programming, habits and impulses. The problem is needed, because at an unconscious level the reptilian/survival or hindbrain feels or perceives safety, even if the reverse is real.

On one level, do some women "need" cancer to give themselves a break? Sadly, I believe the answer is, "Yes, even if it kills them."

It's like having faulty wiring in a fuse box. If a fuse is blown, changing the light globe or turning on the light switch won't have any effect, because you're treating the symptom rather than the origin of the problem. So for instance, starting a diet won't be effective. As the unconscious mind is more powerful than the conscious mind, in an attempt to manage the untreated anxiety, people addiction swap or create clever sabotage patterns. The conscious mind only thinks it's running the show.

When you undergo psychological reversal on an issue, you can quickly become conscious of the unconscious need being met. Only then can the new behaviour be integrated healthily.

I've known many people who've been to various doctors, psychotherapists or counsellors, sometimes for years, without any actual change occurring. Describing problems without giving thought to outcome is like having a headache and asking a bottle of aspirin to cure you. If you want actual change you must become aware of your limiting beliefs and how they're affecting your life. The mind plays the movie that is the projection of your thoughts. Your thoughts are created and believed according to your level of consciousness.

A classic example is why New Year's resolutions generally go in one year and out the other.

### What's your most inspiring client story?

That's such a difficult question. I've been blessed to work with so many beautiful souls. I've been honoured to hear stories of courage, humanity and love. Some have great outcomes and some not so good, as often clients come to me as a last port of call when they may have been unwell for years, have endured lengthy drug regimens or multiple operations and simply don't have enough vital force required to engage in a healing process.

For instance, I met with a lovely woman a few days before she died. Her friend had wanted her to see me months before, but she hadn't been interested in exploring alternative medicine. She was angry about her situation. She had uterine cancer and in her words "did everything" her specialist recommended, but eighteen months later the cancer had returned, and she'd lost the battle. She was unable to accept that she'd come to the end of the road.

We began with a grounding meditation and then emotional freedom release to try to alleviate some of her dreadful discomfort, including extreme nausea. We were tapping together on meridian endpoints and exploring emotions and feelings, when unexpectedly she cried out, "I know what this is about. It's about guilt!" She then went on to tell me about her guilty secret. She'd had a child out of wedlock and had told no one. Decades later, when her family found out about it the same time as her marriage collapsed, it had caused a rupture with one of her children, and she felt the breakdown of her family. "Why didn't my specialist explain this to me?" she pleaded.

In stark contrast, I recently worked with a beautiful lady regarding unwanted weight gain. One of the things I love most about my work is assisting people to come up with their own rituals that work for them on a psychic/ spiritual healing level. During the course of her initial consultation, she shared with me that many years previously she had undergone a double mastectomy. She *knew* she should be grateful to be alive, but she still mourned for her breasts and grieved for her perceived loss of womanhood.

The preparation for her ordeal began when her surgeon entered her hospital room and stated, "You have cancer. Tomorrow we're going to remove your breasts. We're saving your life, so you should be grateful." Then he turned and walked out. I have no doubt that doctors are deeply in need of neuro-emotional healing, as well as the police force and social workers.

The client and I spoke at length about her life and hobbies, among them gardening, knitting and crochet. I assured her on an energetic level she was still perfectly whole and complete, and she could honour that wholeness daily. Then we did some written affirmations around self-love.

Her garden was also a great comfort, so I asked her if she'd placed a tree or shrub of some significance in it. She said she'd planted something special after her mother passed away. I advised her to crochet whatever felt meaningful to her in relation to her breasts. For instance, something representative of a breast, a pouch or circle. She could make it any colour she chose and decorate it any way she saw fit. Then she needed to write herself a love letter, reminding herself of how beautiful she was as a person, friend, daughter, mother and wife, and to wrap the letter in whatever she created and bury it by the bush she'd planted for her mother. She did, and finally, more than two decades after losing a significant part of herself, she gave herself permission to grieve and honour the part thought lost to her.

It was quite remarkable that carrying such deep sadness hadn't created more cancer for her. People are such microcosms in a macrocosm. Her gardening and creativity no doubt saved her. After more than two decades and having lost a significant part of herself, she finally became, to use a Jungian term, *re-membered*. An entirely different person walked into my office the next time. She was so light-hearted. All of the energy that had gone into suppressing grief and sorrow was available to radiate love. We both shed tears of joy together, which is not an unusual occurrence in my work.

I have to say that having experienced several inexplicable spirit-filled happenings personally, and hearing firsthand many stories of miracles, I'm sure death is an awakening and a renewal, a return to the Love-Light Energy Form. I have no doubt we simply shuffle off from our spent physical body, and while I've moved beyond the Christian ideal of Heaven from my childhood, I'm certain we go to a higher spiritual plane. A place of absolute peace and love. And even if loved ones are no longer with us on the earthly plane, there's no separation. They reside forever in the heart and spirit.

And as my own journey with my breast problem? I was lucky enough to check into a five-day solitary retreat. I ate organic food, meditated, relaxed, prayed, read, rested, performed yoga, received several massages and drank a blood-cleansing herbal tea. I endeavoured to take better care of myself, and even though I still had swollen, painful breast lumps for over six months, I stayed positive and was confident of a resolution. One night months later, after meditating deeply, I had a special dream that was so powerful it's stayed with me ever since, and I knew I would be perfectly all right no matter what. My breast lumps mostly resolved within the month afterward. To this day, if ever I get off track, Lefty, my physical-spiritual barometer, aches and reminds me to love and look after myself!

I would like to end with a poem I found years ago. I still endeavour to read it daily as it's immensely powerful. I've bought several copies of

Marianne Williamson's book, *A Return to Love*. I always seem to pay it forward and give it away while reading it, so I never get to the end. It's a gleaming and beautiful pebble to come across on the path of life.

Our deepest fear is not that we are inadequate.

Our deepest fear is that we are powerful beyond measure.

It is our light, not our darkness, that most frightens us.

We ask ourselves, Who am I to be brilliant, gorgeous, talented and fabulous?

Actually, who are you not to be?

You are a child of God.

Your playing small does not serve the world.

There's nothing enlightened about shrinking, so that other people won't feel insecure around you.

We are all meant to shine, as children do.

We were born to make manifest the glory of God that is within us.

It's not just in some of us, it's in everyone.

And as we let our light shine, we unconsciously give other people permission to do the same.

As we are liberated from our own fear, our presence automatically liberates others.
*~ Marianne Williamson*

To discover more about how Heather Belle can help you *Elevate Your Health*, visit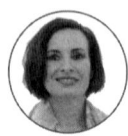

www.elevate-books.com/health

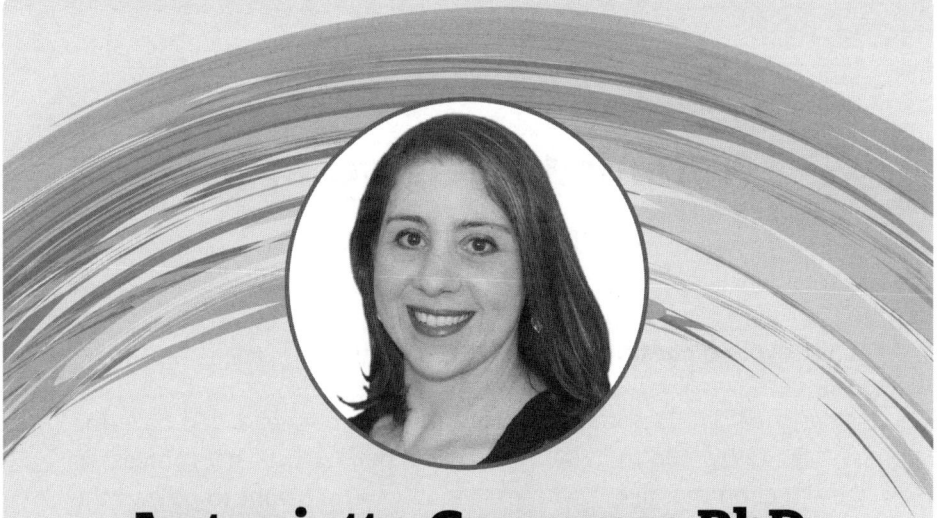

# Antonietta Genovese PhD

## Hear Your Heart's Call

Antonietta Genovese is a certified coach and mentor who holds a PhD in Material Science and First Class Honours, and a B.App.Sc. in Applied Chemistry. Her contribution to collaborative projects that link academia, research organisations and commercial partners, has made her the recipient of the Business-Higher Education Round Table Award (B-HERT), CRC Chairman's awarded for Excellence in Commercialisation and the CRC Association Excellence in Innovation Award. Antonietta has supervised and mentored postgraduate and undergraduate students. She was also actively involved in leading-edge innovative research and development of patented passive fire protection and biodegradable starch packaging materials.

Inspired by a change in focus and a self-initiated project, Antonietta diversified into the area of health and wellness. This led to a growing interest in mindset strategies and personal development and becoming an EDISC consultant. She's always had a passion to help people and continues to inspire through her own example by assisting others to engage, grow and achieve a vibrant life.

# Antonietta Genovese PhD

## Hear Your Heart's Call

### *What's your biggest life lesson?*

My greatest life lesson has been to listen to my heart and have the courage to be true to myself. To make a decision, set my compass in the direction that aligns with my vision of who I want to be and the feelings I desire to experience, and then take the steps to progress forward.

It's about trusting myself as I go into the unknown and opening up to the possibility of creating a life greater than myself and who I'll become. I've been through darkness, and yet amongst those times I've also experienced the sunshine.

My journey is to learn to listen to my heart. If I didn't take the steps to steer into a new direction and create a new path, then I would have followed one that no longer supported my personal growth and experiences. It was up to me to decide to consciously create change in the area of personal health and vitality.

This meant a new beginning. A time to take the steps, one by one, to navigate towards my vision and create a new path to achievement, fulfilment and a deeper level of happiness.

By not listening to your heart, you forfeit the opportunity to evolve and create what you desire deep within yourself. Years will pass, and you will wonder, *What if I took that path instead? What would have happened, and where would I be? How much would I have grown as a person who is capable, knowledgeable, creative and able to go beyond self-imposed limits?*

Everyone has a journey and mission in their current time, space and environment. They can take steps, no matter how small, to move on to something more meaningful and create a life of greater fulfilment for themselves and others.

**What was a major decision you made about your life, and what was the journey you took to get there?**

The major decision was to leave, at least for a while, a world that was a significant part of my life, which was education. After college, I attended university where I completed a First-Class Honours Degree. From there I received an APA Scholarship to pursue my PhD in Material Science and proceeded as a postdoctoral research fellow. I spent my research time developing leading-edge fire retardant and biopolymer composite materials in collaborative research projects.

During this chapter in my life, I couldn't see beyond where I wanted to be or what I wanted to do. I didn't know what my life's purpose was. Attempting to answer questions as to where I would head to next brought on a depth of sadness, because I was unsure how to answer the longer term vision and direction.

Two years before I left, I made an important decision I kept to myself, because I believed no one would understand. I'd decided to change my life and pay more attention to my health and wellbeing. I could no longer continue neglecting what was important to me. An internal calling was incrementally building in amongst the whirlwind of the work and achievements in which I was focused. My job as a researcher consumed me, and this led to more time alone and a sense of disconnection, even when surrounded by work and people every day. Gradually, my inner light dwindled. My spark, fascination and brightness were barely there, and it was reflected in my health. I'd placed a pause button on my life for far too long.

I couldn't remain in academia, at least for the time being. I was offered a research and development position, but a more powerful voice spoke to me. It told me it was time to take care of myself and improve my life through focusing on the health of my mind, body and inner happiness. I decided to listen to my inner voice and have the courage to fly or fall, whatever the path I chose to take, because it was mine to create.

If I'd stayed along the same path, I wouldn't have had many of the new experiences that came to pass. I'm so grateful I made the decision to create the changes that have steered me in a more positive direction of greater fulfilment.

### Why is health important?

The human body is an extraordinary, intricate machine. It can tolerate so much, and ultimately the more you practice activities that lead to ill health, the more it becomes unable to do what it's been designed to do, which is to naturally and effortlessly maintain an optimal state of health and vitality.

My studies and work were the priority above all else in my life and certainly above my health. That final year, the beginning of winter brought on a cough that persisted for way longer than it should, but I didn't let it stop me from the work that needed to be done. I ignored what it was telling me, along with many other warning signs I'd experienced prior. Eventually, I became ill from an infection in my left leg that resulted in pain and an inability to walk.

In addition, I had a significantly larger build and wasn't comfortable in my own skin. Many words are used to describe such a state of physicality that I haven't wanted to hear or say, because of all of the pain, disconnection and isolation I've felt in the past. It was a burden that brought on taunting and teasing. I couldn't look at my reflection and smile, because of the negative self-talk and thoughts that consumed me. This impacted my self-image, self-esteem and self-confidence and hindered me from pursuing many activities in which I desired to partake.

From this aspect, I believe health is vitally important. It impacts vibrancy, vitality and vision. Health is a cornerstone to living, enjoying life, creating happiness within and celebrating with others. Pay attention to what your body tells you. Don't ignore the warning signs, or it could wind up being too late. Prevention is better than a cure later down the track.

Since creating a significant change in my own life in pursuit of a healthier way of living, I've opened doors that once were locked. I've learned it's possible, at any age, to make small changes that radiate out in subtle ways like increased energy, stamina, clarity, focus and creativity.

### What got you interested in health and wellness?

I'd had enough of feeling like I was trapped within a body that didn't represent the true essence of who I was. Underneath the surface, I'd known there was more to life than routine and working within limits. I wanted to break free of the cycle. The numbness of the day-to-day thoughts and busyness. I no longer felt inner joy. Days became mechanical, and I dreaded catching the train, crossing the street and walking up those three polished steps into my workplace. It was like the air became so dense it was challenging to breathe.

I diverted my attention towards questions that fuelled my interest in health and wellbeing. Like when I take on a new research project, there was energy and flow in that direction. My intention kept me going as I gained knowledge that would assist my endeavour. There were elements of fun and a range of emotions to experience that would come with a long-term plan and its execution. I prepared my mind for what was to evolve into my journey.

While in the labs, I asked myself, *How can I get out of this and acquire the time, energy and focus to dedicate to creating a difference and improving my health? How can I give this a real go and recognise sustainable results for the long-term benefits? How can I create a lifestyle and a sense of ecology for years to come?*

There was a foreseeable application of what had worked for others that I wanted to adopt to make it work for me. In essence, to model what aligned to my own ethics and responsibilities toward my holistic health.

With reference to modelling, I focused on different athletes and others who'd changed their lives in a similar way and elucidated what got them their results. Athletes train consistently, with focus, dedication and attention to detail. They often have a team of people around them that includes coaches and nutritionists. I may not have had a team around me, but I did have a vast array of resources to tap into, due to the ease and availably of information on the internet.

In addition to the different aspects of training, there was the element of nutrition to consider. I took note of what would be intuitively sustainable for the long term. There are no quick fixes when it comes to gaining a sustainable lifestyle change and vision I desired to create. It became a case of bringing different elements together in a way that worked congruently, cohesively and with a little creativity thrown into the mix. It wasn't unlike a multidisciplinary project that involves expertise from various resources, distilled into creating a product, outcome or goal in some form. I had trained and performed how to plan, research, experiment and report results and now applied these skills in a different form.

I needed to take aspects of other plans I could adapt for my own journey, in order to sustain my changes. Modelling and extracting useful, practical approaches has helped to shorten the time period of reaching my goal, but there's still the required testing and measuring, because without this part of the feedback loop, change and progress can't be measured and followed over the longer duration.

When embarking on a path, as with any goal, it's important to keep it simple and tap into aspects that work, and then stick with it until a better method is discovered. Bring the inner trust, wisdom and belief that achieving a significant goal can be attained through inspiration, which is stronger than willpower, because willpower is like a battery. It needs to be recharged, whereas inspiration is breathed from within, and the desire is stronger and more sustainable.

### What are your feelings and experiences of being healthy?

Connecting into the feeling, experience and benefits of being healthy is important as an internal driver. In the beginning, it's about imagining what it would feel like to create and have a healthier heart, a strong, fitter, more mobile body, and in turn increased clarity, creativity, enjoyment, and movement, that all align with being healthy.

Why would someone want to create and experience vibrant health? This aspect opens the mindset and inspiration to move forward and facilitate the attainment of both mind and body on the same path. An integration of head and heart towards congruency. The following questions will provide a portal to unveiling your inner truth.

- For what purpose do you want to change?

- What do you desire to experience in life?

- What experiences do you want to create in your life that you've put on hold?

- What benefits would you obtain by creating a healthier body?

- What legacy do you want to create?

I answered these questions in my exploration to achieving a healthier lifestyle and therefore wound up experiencing health in a way I never had before.

In the first phase of physical and mental transformation, I used brainstorming as a way to create a mind map, so I could connect thoughts in a free-flowing manner. A mind map is like a stream of conscious thoughts that helps you explore deeper, tap into feelings of achieving the vision desired and bring it into the present. The more immersed you become in the feelings, and the more detailed they are, the stronger the pull will be towards closing the gap between where you are and where you desire to be.

A mind map can be adopted in any goal. I've utilised it in my research work many times and found it a versatile and adaptable tool. Starting with a central theme/goal, you begin creating branches outward, allowing thoughts/words/emotions/processes to permeate from your unconscious mind and through to your conscious awareness. Reflecting on those words and thoughts opens possibilities even more.

You can write your thoughts as they come to mind. In a more structured and powerful approach, you can utilise the hierarchy of ideas within a mind map construction. A model is often referred to as *chunking* and is a methodology of expanding your thinking to different levels that span from visionary/abstract/big picture to detailed and specific.

How to apply it from the central theme is to ask questions that move you through the levels. Often the same question can be asked multiple times to connect one thought to the following one, until no further thought comes to mind. For instance, moving upward, the questions to elicit thoughts and feelings could be, but are not limited to, the following:

▸ What purpose will _____ serve?

▸ What is the positive intention of _____?

- What will _____ give me?

- What will achieving _____ mean for me?'

Moving downward, the questions delve into the more specific details of the tasks/actions/steps/information that can guide you towards finding what resources may be required toward fulfilment of your goal. The questions tap into the minutiae of what/who/how/when and where. From there you can explore challenges and ways of moving through them in a holistic and resourceful manner.

At any of these levels, lateral exploration can be elucidated by asking, *What else?* Here you open yourself up to more possibility and choice. This model will facilitate you in developing a comprehensive exploration of your thoughts and activities that will guide you towards creating your vision/goal.

A representation of the mind map in its simplest form is shown in Figure 1. The central thought is *Vibrant Health* with three main branches of MIND, BODY and HAPPINESS. Aspects of the desired feelings, self-empowerment and overall impact it would have on self and others, are embedded in the branches. Specifics encompass the tasks/activities, such as the training and movement (for example, resistance, cardiovascular fitness and challenges), as well as nourishment to support the creation of Vibrant Health. There's a cascade of positive flow from taking consistent, small steps, along with conscious thought, until it becomes a way of living, and then layering new activities, thoughts, and challenges to elevate to the next level of self.

What would your mind map look like? What would it reveal for your next vision/goal for yourself? If you take the steps and begin moving in that direction, where will you be heading? Be open to the possibility, explore, and have the courage to fly and reach farther than you ever thought possible.

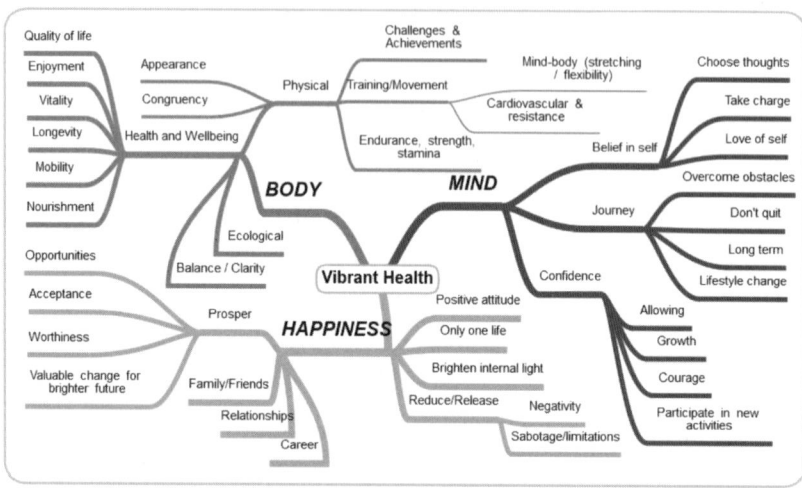

Figure 1: Mind map exploration

## What are the benefits of modern technology, and how do you maintain daily inspiration?

Modern technology has been a great asset, and I've relied on different forms to assist in my journey, specifically to increase my knowledge and learning how to apply it. Utilising my mind map, I had the foundation to direct focus towards searching for information that would assist me through each obstacle or exploration of an idea.

Resources, such as books the internet and experts, are readily available to everyone. There's an array of information that can be tapped into for virtually any area of specificity. In addition, there's software to log programs and monitor change that can be compiled to produce a visual representation of progress. A graph of small successes could be key at times to keep you inspired to keep going. Photographs are another great avenue and one that helped me to see how far I'd gone on my path to health and vitality.

Technology enables access to the latest research and the ability to purchase items you couldn't have access to otherwise. The biggest investment I made was a commercial grade cross-trainer. It became my lifesaver, and I'm grateful for every pedal and hour I've spent improving and maintaining my cardiovascular system, endurance and baseline strength. Part of the decision-making process was to compare specifications of similar cross-trainers and find the ones that suited my intention and requirements. For example, the ergonomic elliptical stride, angle of incline and resistance, and being low impact, while creating a variety of challenges, were important considerations.

Technology has assisted in the feedback cycle on a short, medium and longer-term basis, analogous to working towards milestones of any project. By logging training sessions, appropriate data can be reviewed at intervals to gauge progress and successes. Considering my journey was for long-term, sustainable change, these details were important, especially when I didn't perceive any change through numbers and chose to believe my strength and endurance were increasing. The thought of the dreaded plateau can play mind games at times, so the reminder of the big picture, the inspiration, the vibrant health, and all of the eventual benefits, were what moved me through, as challenging as many of those days were.

If you don't document some form of measurement, then it can be difficult to trace progress. A feeling of progress supports inner happiness.

**What strategies have you used and maintained to keep you on track to a more balanced life?**

One facet of my mentality that contributed toward my success was how I structured my day, week and month with anchor points that were dedicated towards my training routine. They became a ritual that remains a consistent and valued part of my life, health and vitality.

Creating a structured routine gave my mind focus for the days ahead, even when I had unwanted thoughts. Training comprised both cardiovascular and resistance aspects, with their own inherent challenges that kept me occupied as I recorded progress, whether it was a time extension, increased resistance, reduced resting heart rate, or faster heart rate recovery. The more I improved my cardiovascular fitness, the greater the endurance and the higher the resistance I could maintain.

As my self-image and confidence improved, and I reached a personal milestone, I joined a local gym. To have the courage to even step into a gym was a significant step. I had the perception you had to already be fit and look great, but I was wrong. Going to the gym not only extended my skills but got me to connect with more people and create another level of balance.

My efforts were richly rewarded. I met some wonderful ladies of all ages and fitness levels, who were supportive and encouraging. Later that year there was a farewell gathering on a Friday evening for a trainer at the gym, where I was asked if I would like to do a 14km Fun Run that Sunday. Thoughts churned in my mind of the hours spent clocking 10km consistently on my cross-trainer and the trust I'd built up in my endurance. How would I handle an additional 4km? Instinctively, I decided to do it. To be truthful, only two weeks prior I'd run 2km nonstop for the first time. I remember the sensation of calmness. A kind of certainty that what I was about to embark on what was going to be a test of how far I'd progressed.

The morning of the run, I met up with a fellow runner, and we championed each other. We agreed to jog together and whenever we separated along the route, we would just keep going. We kept a fairly even pace from the starting line to about the 3km mark. At that point we ran our own race, and I headed on, knowing we would meet at the end.

I hadn't realised how long 14km really was and how challenging running on a concrete road would be. My sneakers were nothing fancy, so I trusted my stride, pace and breathing. I began to play games in my mind. A strategy that kept me moving forward was keeping pace with a runner a little ahead of me and sometimes breaking into a small sprint.

I counted the kilometres one by one. By the eighth or ninth kilometre, I felt exhausted, my feet were sore and I wanted to stop for a rest. But I knew if I stopped, I wouldn't be able to keep going, so I jogged a little slower. Not once did I stop or slow to a walk.

I knew I was approaching the finish line. The fresh air along Beach Road, St Kilda, was welcoming. During the last couple of kilometres, I was surprised to see the back of someone I felt was more of a runner than I was. I tapped her on the shoulder and said hello for the briefest moment, before I kept going with a smile on my face, knowing that if I went as fast as I could, I would cross that finish line with a time to be proud of. Heart pumping, feet hurting, I managed to conjure enough energy to cross that finish line. Music blared, people cheered and I smiled from ear to ear. It was the most exhilarating feeling I'd ever felt. It was like I was flying. It's the kind of freedom that mobility gives, and I will never forget it. I wouldn't have thought I could accomplish running nonstop. In the end, my time was a proud 1:28:48.

This was one of my happiest, proudest moments. I overcame many limitations. It was a summation of all of the steps I'd taken to improve my health and fitness. I trusted my mind and body to run the distance and believed in myself and my capacity. Without achieving a sustainable and manageable way of living, I wouldn't have been able to accomplish this feat, let alone other runs I've completed since.

Sometimes events like this can challenge you and show you the resilience, determination and resolve you have within yourself. I utilised the same attributes as I had for accomplishing many academic achievements, but this one gave me a sense of freedom on a personal level.

### How does someone make the choice to step into happiness?

Creating greater levels of happiness within yourself raises the foundational level overall within your body and contributes to your health and wellbeing. Happiness comes from your own choice to be happy. Honour and be true to yourself by creating experiences that nurture and build on that foundational level of happiness. It's within your own power to choose to be happy now, no matter how long the journey.

Not only do I feel younger, there's a sense of liberation and light-heartedness that comes with the removal of a heavy burden. Transformation to a state of health and vitality requires the integration of mindset, nutrition and movement into creating harmony and happiness within, and that balance is reflected outward.

The more I changed and understood the feedback loop, the more I came to appreciate the strength and beauty within, and allowed it to radiate out into the world. Of course, I have my moments when it dims, because that's part of the human condition. The difference now is that I can turn it back on much faster.

Overall, after experiencing the shift in my own energy and presence, I've opened doors to experiences I'd previously locked away and stepped into a new space of expansion and growth. There's a greater drive to move forward from a place of calmness, love and connection.

Connecting the mind as an extension of the heart, while nurturing creativity and power, is where harmony brings together the fruition of what you desire. By becoming more in flow and attentive to what makes you feel good, it allows growth and prosperity to fill you deeply, and through the utilisation of your power of creation, you can express more of who you truly are.

### What was your biggest fear, and how did you overcome it?

I don't think you can really overcome fear, but you can turn it into familiarity. Fear is within you to protect you and comes from an evolutionary origin. It can be viewed as a doorway to an exciting opportunity yet to be embraced, and provide fuel for growth and change.

During the past year, I've challenged myself to have new experiences that would lead to significant milestones of change and personal growth. One of those experiences was travelling on my own, as previously I had only travelled with others. I organised all of the details and trusted I would be okay. Even though it was interstate, it was an adventure, and I felt a sense of freedom and mobility. I travelled to the beautiful Narrabeen, a suburb outside of Sydney, for a short stay to attend a workshop. I went a few days earlier, as I decided to see the sights and participate in some activities beforehand. I'd planned to climb the Sydney Harbour Bridge, which had been a goal of mine for some time.

The day after I arrived, I caught the bus to town and spent a while getting lost in the streets looking for the bridge walk entrance. I had a moment of thinking, *What am I doing here all on my own, with no one to talk to?* A sense of panic came over me. I had two close friends a phone call away. If I didn't find that entrance, I was going to give up.

After taking a few deep breaths, I centred myself and had the courage to continue. I got my bearings with a map and found the entrance. I'd already climbed the bridge in my mind, yet I had a mixture of feelings leading up to the climb itself. I walked to the counter and asked the young gentleman to describe the climbs and safety precautions, but I don't think I was listening to his answer, because the adrenaline was already pumping.

I had chosen to climb the uppermost part of the bridge, since I was going to immerse myself into the full Sydney Harbour Bridge experience. Before going on the bridge, each participant in the group openly shared their reason for being there. Once the pre-safety training was done, we were asked who was most afraid, and I rapidly put up my hand, so I wound up first in line to climb the bridge. It meant I would be the leader.

The most challenging part was climbing up four sets of steep stairs. The rest was a breeze. We had the most beautiful day, and with the clear sky, I could see for miles. I knew I'd experienced something special that day, so afterward I made my way to the harbour and relaxed. I captured the moment, and in essence my broader transformational journey, in the following poem.

### A Moment's Stillness on the Bridge

*So, I take a chance,*
*Wondering, contemplation, exhilaration.*
*What might it be for me?*
*Opportunity to step beyond, with anticipation.*

*So, I step through the door,*
*The one that appeared before me, right there on the wall,*
*The other side is the call,*
*For it is I that must have courage to fly or fall.*

*The voice within, whispers in my ear,*
*The voice within, listen to it and hear,*
*The thoughts that say, this is the way,*
*The thoughts that say, let go, embrace your fear for today.*

*So, I step out on the bridge,*
*The platform below supports my feet,*
*Only one way to go,*
*Trust myself, and let it really show!*

*One by one, step by step,*
*Thought by thought, breath by breath,*
*Heart sings, beat by beat,*
*Mind wins, the summit I'll greet!*

*Along the climb, a moment met,*
*When all stood still, a pause I kept,*
*All the sounds just disappeared,*
*In that moment, nothing I feared.*

*As one, with the breeze of the air,*
*As one, with the water below,*
*As one, with the resonance of the bridge,*
*As one, in harmony and flow.*

*Stillness, within my mind,*
*Stillness, within my thoughts,*
*Flags flutter with the winds above,*
*Surrounding space, light and love.*

*The moment ends,*
*I move on,*
*And up the steps,*
*New thoughts dawn.*

*The bridge I know, that I can climb,*
*The other side, there is more to find,*
*What awaits, I will face,*
*With wonder and awe, curiosity and grace.*

**How are you making a difference in people's lives?**

During each stage of my life, the core essence to assist and make a difference has prevailed. I do it through guidance, mentoring, demonstrating or enlightening conversation. Having spent so much time in academia, I've assisted and contributed on many levels with peers, fellow researchers and students in collaborative, multidisciplinary teams.

It's through my experience and learning that I'm now able to appreciate and assist others in their journey. As a certified coach and mentor, I facilitate clients through their challenges, so they can cross their bridge toward their vision. It truly starts with honouring and loving yourself and recognising you matter. Have the courage to take that first step, knowing you have the choice to create a more vibrant life, one with greater love, joy and harmony.

### How did you become your own success story?

My mentor, Sherryn Bowers, shared an insight with me, which is, "When you go through greater depths of pain, it opens you to greater heights of love, joy, passion and life." This can be in any area. An important aspect is to be an observer and find the gems, while experiencing the depths. These represent learnings. Notice attributes that were harnessed in those times and the strength you had to move through them. Appreciate and find ways to be grateful for them. The experiences, learning and achievements I had during my time at university have shown me who I am, as well as the courage, resilience and determination to accomplish my goals.

You can use the power of appreciation and gratitude to inspire yourself to create change. Through believing, trusting and acknowledging where you are and infusing it with love and light, you can transform and radiate even brighter. Liberate that true essence of you by writing your own life story with that golden pen, because you're certainly worth it!

 To discover more about how Antonietta can help you *Elevate Your Health*, visit

www.elevate-books.com/health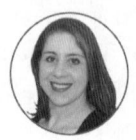

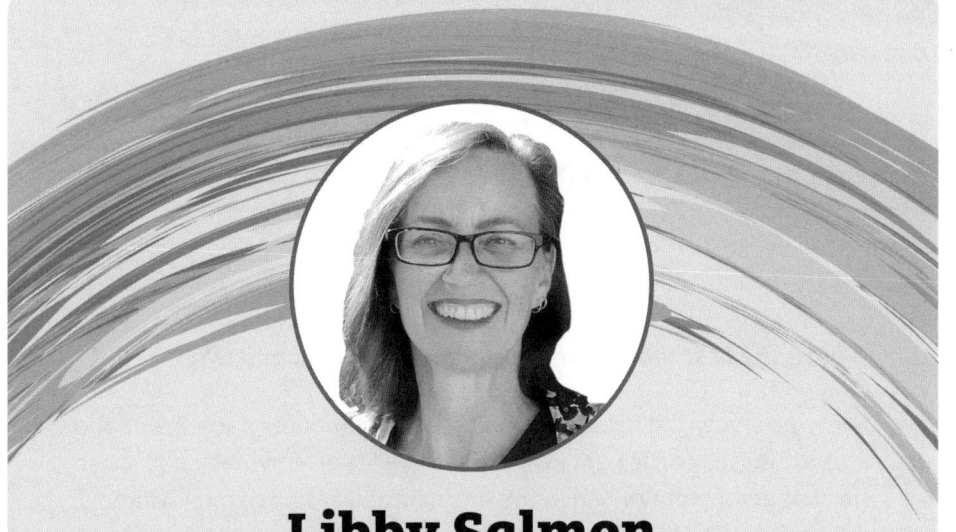

# Libby Salmon

## Cellular Communication

Compelled to find ways of preventing injury to maintain her active daughter's health and wellbeing during a competitive, and then professional, ice skating career, Libby utilised a variety of different methods, including many forms of Western medicine, only to realise they were temporary.

After sourcing a number of products, Libby discovered self-controlled energo-adaptive-regulator (SCENAR) technology and eventually became a SCENAR Therapist.

Now Libby operates her business, Bio Circuitry, and distributes a range of products that interact with the body's electrical system to promote health and wellbeing. She is proficient in the use of all of her products and provides a high level of caring customer support to her clients. Libby's goal is to help everyone become pain-free while maintaining an active lifestyle.

# Libby Salmon
## Cellular Communication

***What's the best thing that ever happened to you and why?***

My twelve-year-old daughter, Elinor, was a competitive ice skater and an enthusiastic participant in an exhaustive list of activities, so much so she was getting out of bed in the morning and saying to me, "Mummy, my legs hurt." The pain wasn't so bad that she stopped any of her activities, so I was slow to realise there was an actual problem. I'll admit it wasn't one of my finer parenting moments.

When I finally did catch on, I started massaging Elinor's legs each evening in an effort to release the muscles. When that didn't work, I took her to massage therapists, physiotherapists and the local GP with little result, because she would continue to launch herself into the world each day and reverse any progress that had been made.

Then a friend of mine mentioned SCENAR to me, which is a Self-Controlled-Energo-Adaptive-Regulator. There's a lot of science behind it, so I'll keep the technical jargon to a minimum, but basically it's an electro-therapeutic device used to deliver pain relief and restore function. It sets up a two-way communication with the nervous system and encourages it to redirect its activity towards areas of weakness in the body.

By this time I had attempted a number of "mainstream" solutions, so I thought we would give it a try. After all, it was drug free, non-invasive, and painless. What did we have to lose? I took Elinor along for a session, and I have to say the transformation was incredible. There really is no other word to describe it. She went from complaining that it hurt to walk to increasing the size of her skating jumps by almost thirty centimetres after just one session!

Elevate Your Health

Needless to say, I was intrigued. I took Elinor back for a second therapy session the following week just to check, even though she seemed fine and had no pain in her legs.

Pretty soon after that I bought my first personal interactive neuro-feedback device called an ENAR, which was a copy of the SCENAR. It cost a small fortune, and personal SCENAR devices were not available in Australia at the time.

I used the ENAR on family and friends and got some pretty good results, considering I really had no idea what I was doing or what was going on. The only drawback was that the signal was a bit *bitey*, and some people didn't like the feel of it. Nor did I, so I never really used it much for any of my own small aches and pains. I still have that device, and it still works, but I have other, better devices now.

Some time between six months and a year later, the price of the professional devices dropped, and I bought my very first professional SCENAR. Then I enrolled in Level 1 SCENAR training.

I had no intention to go any further than understanding the technology and use it to treat family and friends. I found the whole thing fascinating and wanted to learn as much as I could.

This training changed my life. Okay, so maybe there were a few other factors and more learning, but this was the start. The Level 1 SCENAR training, as it was then, went through the basic principles and protocols of the device and how to best work with it. This was an eye-opening experience, because apart from having had the occasional massage and knowing acupuncture and Chinese medicine existed, I was mainstream Western medicine all the way. I didn't believe in *a pill for every ill*, but I had never considered there were other ways of working with the body to improve overall wellbeing and deliver pain relief. In my defence, I've been fortunate enough to not have experienced pain or ill health in the way I know many people have, so I hadn't been looking, either.

The SCENAR device and technology was developed in Russia, and a large part of the philosophy behind the SCENAR protocols is drawn from Traditional Chinese Medicine (TCM) and an associated understanding of energy medicine. The Russians have their own take on medicine as well, and although many of their systems are becoming westernised, I believe the Russian culture has played a large part in developing the classical SCENAR protocols.

SCENAR therapy is all about working with local zones. These are point-of-pain techniques and general zones, which are ways to affect the body in a more *wholistic* manner to improve general wellbeing and outcomes for chronic conditions by working through the nervous system.

If you have a personal SCENAR, ENAR, or other device that uses SCENAR technology, you can download "Basic Steps to Getting the Most from Your Personal SCENAR Device" from http://biocircuitry.com.au/free-basic-scenar-use-download/.

Over the years, since my first encounter with SCENAR and from learning as much as possible to do with the technology, the body's electrical system, and from talking with other therapists, my opinion is that a large part of the success of SCENAR therapy is due to improved cell communication.

### How can cell communication be affected in the body?

The body has an electrical system people pretty much ignore. Sure, if you ask, some might say that the nervous system, heart, and brain are electrical, but they don't *think* about the body being electrical, and many don't take this into consideration at all.

Every cell in the body has a charge, and every thought is an electrical potential. Basically, everyone walks around in their own electromagnetic bio-field and interacts with every other energy source out there, such as the sun, other people, the lights in the room, Wi-Fi...You get the picture. Everything! Robert O. Becker was one of the first scientists to write about this, and if you're at all interested I recommend getting hold of *The Body Electric* as a good starting point.

All of this reading gave me a better understanding of how the body maintains homeostasis (balance) by using cell communication and the way this ultimately assists in how you heal—or not. If you do nothing else but somehow improve the communication between individual cells, you can improve the body's ability to heal. This is because now that the cells can talk with each other, the body knows there's a problem down the line and can send the relevant resources to the damaged area.

So every time someone discovers a new *magic bullet*, or rediscovers an old one, if you exclude pharmaceutical drugs it's likely that when you break it down to basics, it works because it improves cell communication. This can be as simple as improving your diet or water consumption.

### Does improved hydration improve cell communication?

Absolutely! As well as good food, exercise, and sleep.

Good hydration means drinking water and not tea, coffee, soft drinks, cordials, vitamin water or alcohol. It also means good-quality water as well. The body has to work harder to process all of those other additives, whether they're loosely classed as foods or are actual pollutants, so drinking the best-quality water available will help your cells communicate. Even water that may have some additives will usually be a better choice than a soft drink or coffee. You can still have these occasionally, or even an alcoholic drink, just don't do it all of the time, and don't kid yourself that it counts as a form of hydration. Drinks that contain caffeine or alcohol are known as diuretics, which means you lose more fluid than you take in. So if you drink a lot of these, you're dehydrating instead of hydrating.

There's an interesting transcript of a lecture delivered by Dr Fereydoon Batmanghelidj called "The Body's Many Cries for Water" that has to do with dehydration and chronic pain. Dr Batmanghelidj was a political prisoner during the Iranian Revolution and would treat his fellow inmates by instructing them to drink water. An extraordinary number of people recovered from their illnesses and survived, all because they were better hydrated. This is a remarkable story, as well as an incredibly easy and cheap solution that could improve overall wellbeing for many. Dr. Batmanghelidj makes the correlation that if each cell is better hydrated, it means that instead of them looking like a sultana, they more resemble grapes, which in turn means the cells are better able to communicate and reduce overall stress.

Dr Batmanghelidj is not alone in this belief. Through the ages water has been proposed as a cure, and there have been several books written on the subject from many parts of the world.

### What part does good food play in cell communication?

An enormous amount! In the words of Michael Pollan in his book *In Defence of Food*, "Eat food, mostly green, not too much." This pretty much rules out most of what's sold as food in supermarkets. It's also a commentary on portion sizes sold in takeaway food restaurants.

Most food today is not really nutritious, and in my opinion you have to be suspicious of anything that can be kept out of the fridge without worrying about it spoiling. Those cheese products not kept in the cold section, for example.

So the first, and most difficult, task is to identify what is *good* food. The easiest way to do this is to put all processed food into the *not good* pile and cook your own. I can hear you groaning about how it takes too long to prepare food from scratch, but it doesn't take much longer, really. It does involve some planning, and I think this is where people have become lazy.

If you cook your own food from fresh ingredients, over time you will notice a change in how you're feeling and potentially how much you eat. The reason for this is relatively straightforward. There are more nutrients when you start with fresh ingredients, and there are fewer preservatives, such as sugar and other chemicals.

So by increasing the quality of the nutrients and reducing the number of chemicals you're consuming, your body is better able to process what you eat, which indirectly results in improved cell communication.

If preparing meals from fresh ingredients is a stretch for you, then even just reading the labels on the food you're buying can allow you to make better, more informed choices, which on its own can result in better cell communication.

### What are some actions people can take to maintain good cell communication?

### Exercise

Exercise is another factor in cell communication, and this can be as simple as just getting your blood moving. Find something that works for you. People's lives today are largely sedentary, so they don't move as much as they should. I'm no expert, but I can say that exercise indirectly helps cell communication by moving nutrients and oxygen around the body and removes toxins.

### Sleep

Sleep is important when it comes to cell communication. And it's not just about quantity but also quality.

When you sleep, you heal. Your grandmother was right! There's an enormous amount of repair work and processing that takes place while sleeping occurs, and much of it doesn't even start until you've been asleep for two to three hours.

At that point, there's a hormone cascade that starts with melatonin from the pineal gland and results in the release of an extraordinary number of hormones from the pituitary and hypothalamus, which are integral to the body's ability to repair itself. So if you mess up the original release of melatonin, you end up affecting the hormonal messaging of your entire system. If this disrupted hormonal messaging becomes chronic, it can result in any number of conditions related to hormonal imbalance.

The pineal gland is affected by light, and it's involved in regulating your biological clock. The bad news is that the advent of electricity has had a negative effect on this process. With the day/night movement of the earth around the sun, at the end of each day the setting of the sun changes the light to a red base. This is an indicator to the pineal gland that night is coming, and it should start preparing for the increased release of melatonin once you go to sleep.

Because most electric light, including computer screens, televisions, tablets and phones have a blue-based background, the pineal gland doesn't receive any preparatory messaging that you're soon going to sleep. This means that when you do get into bed your brain is still buzzing, and you find it difficult to go to sleep. It also means it will take about two to three hours of sleep before you're able to start releasing the necessary increased levels of melatonin.

The other really big factor many people aren't aware of is that if you wake up in the middle of the night and turn on a light or look at your phone, the white light interrupts the production of melatonin, and you have to start all over again. So the quality of your sleep is poor, and you feel tired when you wake in the morning. Your body also hasn't had the time to carry out the necessary repair processes, which can compound if you don't change your habits.

Of course, there may be other health factors involved. However, there are some fairly simple and cheap ways to help change the way you manage the end of your day in order to help improve sleep quality.

▸ Change light globes in your home to have a red base instead of a blue base. The blue-based light globes are usually called something like *bright white* or *cool*, and the red-based ones are *warm* or *natural*. There are new globes and lamps being developed all of the time and some you can program to adjust to your own time zone. The difference is subtle but can have a big impact on your sleep. Pay particular attention to the light globes in bedside lamps and in the rooms you spend time in at the end of the day.

▸ If you or your child needs a nightlight, choose one with a red globe. It won't interrupt the production of melatonin when you wake through the night, which means getting back to sleep will be easier.

▸ Find add-on apps for your electronic gadgets that change the background to a red base. f.lux is one I use and can be found at https://justgetflux.com/. There are others around, so do your research and find one that's suitable for your application.

▸ You could just stop using your computers and gadgets in the evenings. I know this is a bit radical for some people and totally impractical for others. At least set yourself a time after which you won't use your phone or computer, and see how your body adapts.

### Does stress affect cell communication?

Yes, any stress on the body elicits a response. In many cases this is fine, since the body is doing what it's supposed to. It's when the stress situation becomes chronic that problems occur, and the body starts to exhibit signs of exhaustion. As part of my anatomy and physiology studies, I was required to write an essay. I chose to write about chronic stress. The choice was deliberate at the time, because I had an understanding by then that a lot of chronic illness or pain is the result of chronic stress, and I wanted to understand more about it.

The modern lifestyle doesn't give you an opportunity to relax, and in many cases what's thought of as relaxing is just a different kind of stress. Think about playing a computer game as a form of relaxation. You may think of it as fun, because it doesn't relate to work or having to be somewhere. But all of the flashing lights, sounds and storylines are designed to get your adrenaline pumping. They're actually provoking a number of stress responses from the body.

As I read and researched, I discovered that the overloaded stress response, often called adrenal fatigue, in turn resulted in lack of cell communication. This means you can affect the body's stress response and improve its ability to deal with different stressors, physical or mental, by improving cell communication, or vice versa.

### Are there negative effects as a result of using technology?

Yes, and some fairly major ones, too. A few years ago I came across Floww Health Technology. They've produced a technology designed to reduce the effect of non-ionising radiation on the human body. I know. I'm venturing into technological waters again, so my explanation will be brief.

Radiation is divided into ionising and non-ionising radiation. Ionising radiation is emitted by, for instance, X-rays and nuclear power sources and is called *ionising* because the radiation causes the cells it impacts with to lose electrons. This causes the cell to become ionised. That is, the cell now has a positive charge and has been altered as a result of the interaction with the radiation. This kind of radiation has been recognised as damaging for a long time.

*Non-ionising* electromagnetic radiation (EMF or EMR) is the kind of radiation emitted by mobile phones, Wi-Fi, microwaves, hair dryers, electrical wiring in the walls, or basically any electrical device. It doesn't break the electron bonds, so the cell survives the exposure, but there are other biological influences on the cell, such as stress proteins. So while the cell survives, it's still affected by the radiation. If the stress proteins are constantly being activated by exposure to non-ionising radiation, people are essentially living in a state of stress all of the time. The body isn't able to repair itself, because there's no downtime in which to heal. This is recent information, and many people still claim non-ionising radiation is safe.

The problem is that global safety standards have been set using research into the *thermal* effects of EMR, such as when you cook food in a microwave, which is the same kind of radiation your mobile uses to carry out a call.

There's not as much research into the *biological* effects of EMR, which is what should be focussed on. If when you use your phone it warms up the side of your head, this wouldn't be a terribly big problem. But if it changes the cells *inside* of your head, this is a much greater problem. When you pay more attention, you start to see clues. Scientists and researchers have been warning about the biological effects of EMR for some time now.

### What evidence is there that this radiation may be damaging?

In 1971, the U.S. Naval Medical Research Institute published a research document called "Bibliography of Reported Biological Phenomena (Effects) and Clinical Manifestations Attributed to Microwave and Radio-Frequency Radiation" that lists over 2,300 papers and documents regarding the biological effects of non-ionising radiation. The fact that this document was requested by the U.S. Navy in the first place seems to indicate they knew the fields emitted by its radar equipment were causing disease in its crews, and in particular its radar operators.

In the 1970s, Dr. Robert Becker, an American orthopaedic surgeon, was at the forefront of research into electrobiology. He was outspoken about the potential dangers of power lines to human health, but he and his fellow researcher, Dr. Andrew Marino, were largely ignored. Many agree that due to Dr Becker speaking out, his career was affected.

In 1989, the book *Electromagnetic Man: Health and Hazard in the Electrical Environment* was published by Cyril Smith, a retired professor of Electronic and Electrical Engineering at Salford University in England and Simon Best, a medical journalist. It explores the health impact of electromagnetic pollution, chronic exposure to electromagnetic fields and possible solutions.

In 2010, Professor Sam Milham, an American medical epidemiologist, wrote a book called *Dirty Electricity: Electrification and the Diseases of Civilization,* which outlines his concerns and findings regarding the health impacts of electrification. Professor Milham was able to show that the health of humanity has been affected by the introduction of electricity to one degree or another, since its introduction. He's also published several research articles that are available online.

I could go on, but I think I've made my point. The upshot is that because electricity and the resultant technology are so useful, people are busy ignoring the global-scale health impacts.

If this is news to you, I recommend you have a look at the "Bioinitiative Report" (www.bioinitiative.org) and any of the work by Devra Davis, Magda Havas, Dariusz Lesczynski, Olle Johannsen and Martin Blank, to name a few . They're all scientists or doctors speaking out about the dangers of electromagnetic radiation to human health. Microwave News (www.microwavenews.com) and Powerwatch (www. powerwatch.org.uk) are also great online resources.

### What symptoms do people experience as a result of exposure to EMR?

EMR causes stress on the body, and because everybody's stress response is different, the health impacts of EMR exposure are as well. The symptoms people experience can vary wildly from mild to severe, such as headaches and migraines, nausea and chronic digestive issues, and anxiety and depression. Basically any symptom people experience as a result of a stressor can be a symptom of EMR exposure, and currently there's little or no recognition that EMR can affect your health. Symptoms are so general they're often attributed to other sources. The stress caused by EMR is also cumulative, so people can exhibit no symptoms for many years and then develop sensitivity to EMR.

I also believe that like any other stress, often people are able to manage it, and it's not until there are a number of factors occurring at once that cause symptoms to be heightened, that people become sick but are unable to pinpoint the cause.

### Is there a way to combat these symptoms?

This got me thinking. If EMR causes stress, and stress reduces cell communication, what happens if you're somehow able to reduce the effect of EMR from the immediate environment? There's a video on my website that shows what can happen to your blood cells if you're able to reduce the effect of EMR from a mobile phone. You can watch it at www.biocircuitry.com.au/floww-emf-protection/.

There's also a free download that provides information regarding how to reduce your EMR exposure. Most are free and easy to implement. You can find them at http://biocircuitry.com.au/free-reduce-radiation-download. To a certain extent, this document is about turning off gadgets at the source and thinking about the bigger impact of your actions, such as where you carry or leave your mobile phone.

There are also a number of products on the market that transform the immediate environment. I distribute the Floww Health Technology range in Australia, which I believe is one of the best in the field. The simplicity and sophisticated technology, as well as the demonstrated effectiveness, are the reasons I stock them. For more information on these products, visit www.biocircuitry.com.au/floww-emf-protection/the-floww-principle/.

Products that block EMR can also be useful, but you need to think about how you're using them. For example, if you put something on the back of your phone that blocks radiation, your phone will increase its power, in other words its EMR output, in order to get a signal. So you could be increasing your exposure instead of reducing it.

***Despite its harmful effects, do you think technology is useful for communication? Does the good outweigh the bad?***

I love technology, and I am a bit of a geek, but I think people don't always manage it too well, and it's starting to use us instead of us using it.

In this fast-paced, techno-driven world, people have been led to believe that the newest gadget will better connect them to friends and family. While this is true at some level, if the communication takes place in online bites or a shared picture or video on social media, that's not really sharing opinions and beliefs. It's the appearance of sharing and connection while hiding behind a mask displayed to the world that's seldom truly honest.

As technology is used more and more for communication, I believe people are losing, or not learning, some of these important skills that are exercised when speaking face-to-face with others.

For example, if you watch a video of someone delivering a seminar or speech instead of being in the room with them, you're not receiving most of the energetic information from that person as they speak about their subject. You're also not experiencing any aromatic clues.

Then if you take away the video component of the seminar, you're left with a voice recording only, and now have no visual clues. If you then read a transcript, you're removing all tonal cues. It's often still possible to have a good idea of the seminar content, but the resultant transcript is not a *wholistic* way to communicate, and the passion and energy of the speaker is lost.

As you watch television or computer video and listen to radio or podcasts, you need to be aware that at some level of consciousness, much of the material has been tailored to suit the purposes of the creator, and by scripting and rehearsing the material, your responses are being manipulated by the producer. Don't get me wrong, I believe this also happens to a degree in live productions.

When you text or email, you also need to bear in mind that your friend or colleague may not read the message in the same vein as it was intended. What may have an element of humour to it when a person can see your facial expression and hear your tone of voice, may sound rude or mean when it's read. How many times have you received an email that at first seemed offensive, but then when you read it again, perhaps when you were in a better mood, you realised it wasn't?

**What do you think are the important factors for good communication?**

Communication needs to be allowed to happen. It needs time to develop as a shared experience and not forced. I feel blessed that when my daughter was young, she chose ice skating as her sport. While I in no way relished getting out of bed at four am to take her to training four mornings a week, it did mean we spent about an hour and a half in the car each time. This was largely before she had a mobile phone, which meant we had all of that time to talk to each other. This is the same as my dad referring to washing up as a social event.

I think as a result, my daughter and I have a strong relationship. We're so brutally honest with each other now, that other people find this level of honesty confronting. It sometimes can be, and when this happens I realise how fortunate we are. I think honesty in communication is important, although I sometimes find other people can be uncomfortable with this level of honesty, so I try to temper it a bit.

I also believe people need to share knowledge and resources more. It's when you become attached to what you know or have, that communication starts to break down. When you try to protect a position by making something exclusive or to maintain your importance, you can limit the benefits to a much wider group of people.

For everyone and the planet to survive, communication needs to take place at every level: cellular, body system, family, community, state, country and global.

### How has your life changed since discovering SCENAR?

That chance encounter with SCENAR has completely changed my life and has allowed me to establish a business that helps people to manage their own pain and wellbeing. It's opened my eyes to different ways of working to improve health and rekindled my love of learning, as well as broadened my thinking.

I believe communication is the beginning, middle and end of any good relationship. If honesty is compromised, then so is the relationship. This holds true in romantic/life partnerships, friendships, business, and politically and globally.

By improving communication at all levels of existence, people are able to elevate their own lives, as well as those they come in contact with. And as this happens, their influence spreads.

I will leave you with this quote. Sadly, I have no idea who John A. Piece was or what else he wrote:

"Communication is not only the essence of being human, but also a vital property of life."
- *John A. Piece*

 To discover more about how Libby can help you *Elevate Your Health*, visit

www.elevate-books.com/health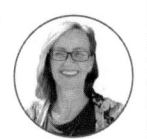

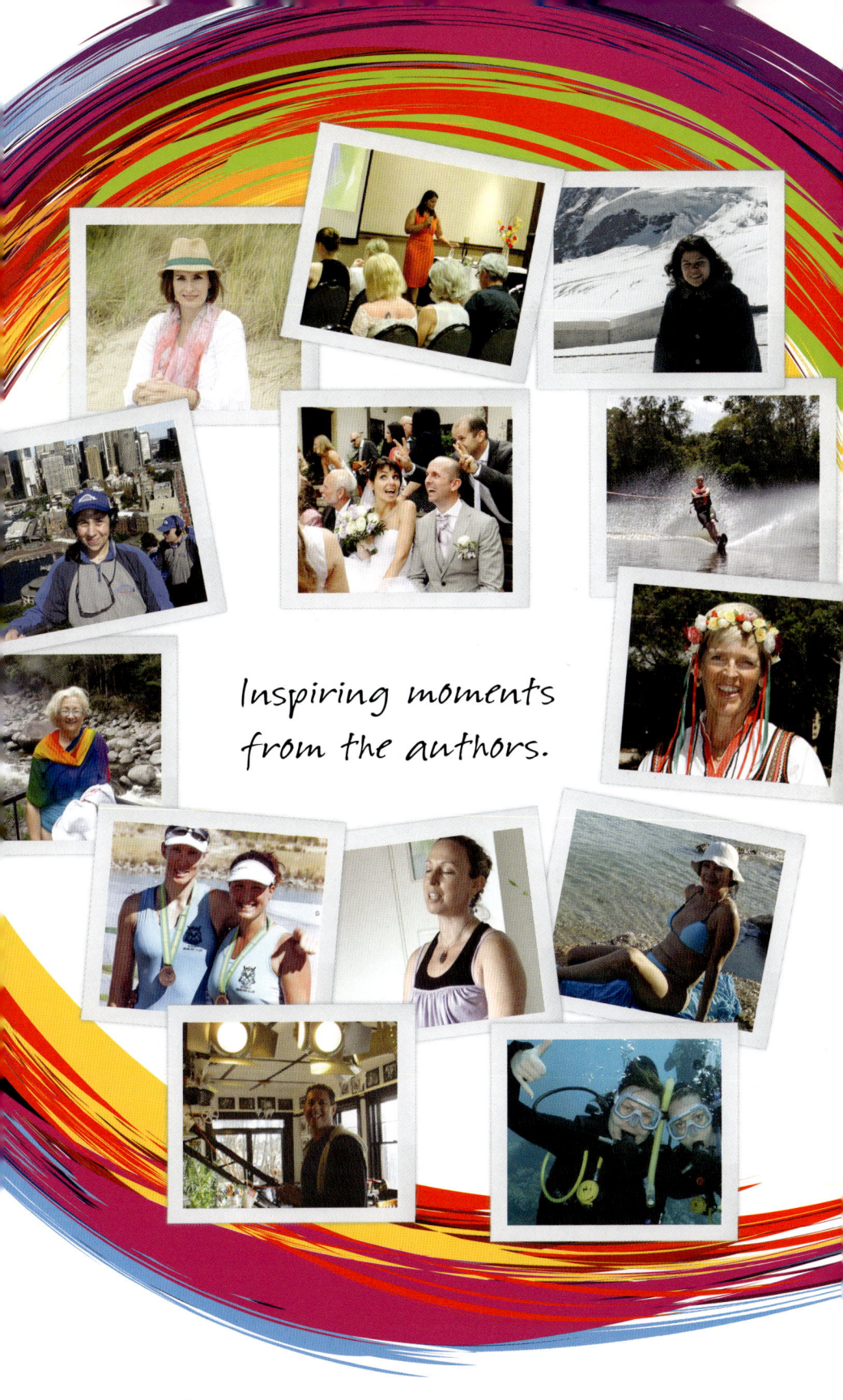

Inspiring moments from the authors.

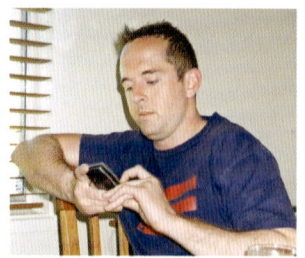
Ben in his "larger" not-so-healthy days.

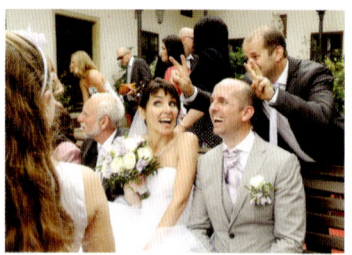
Ben and his wife on their wedding day in a castle in the Czech Republic.

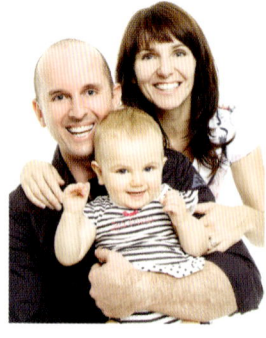
Ben with his wife and daughter.

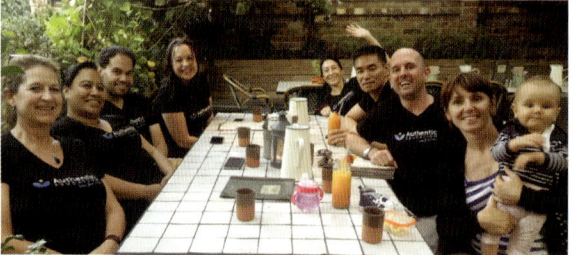
The Authentic Education team sporting their new branded t-shirts, along with team mascot Annabella (Ben's daughter).

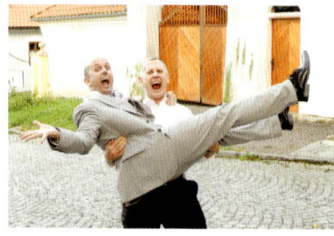
Ben with his Dad.

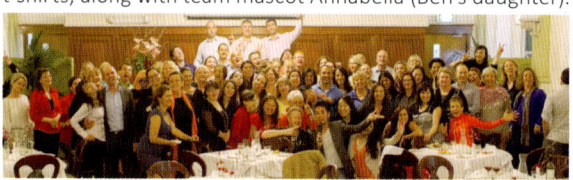
Ben taking his students to dinner upstairs at Authentic Education Academy in Sydney, located inside of a boutique hotel.

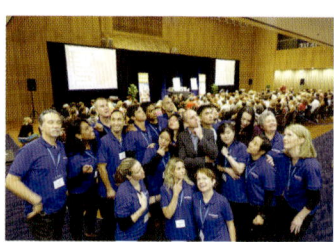
Benjamin Harvey, Cham Tang and Toni Neill (Crew Director and Events Manager), with the crew in blue at an Authentic Education event.

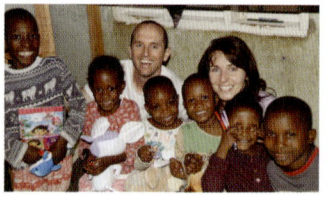
Ben and his wife donating bunk beds and toys at an orphanage in Tanzania.

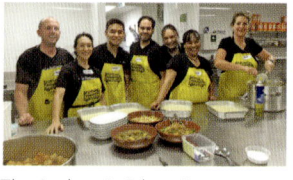
The Authentic Education team (left-right) Ben, Marie, Cham, Raymond, Toni, Eugenie and Kim lending a helping hand at Oz Harvest, the food rescue charity.

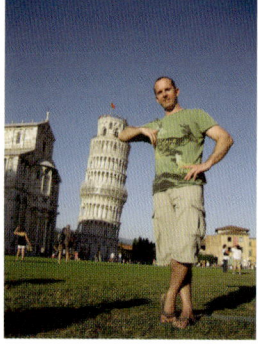
Ben doing the obligatory Leaning Tower of Pisa pose.

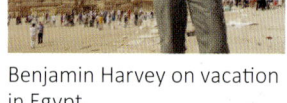
Benjamin Harvey on vacation in Egypt.

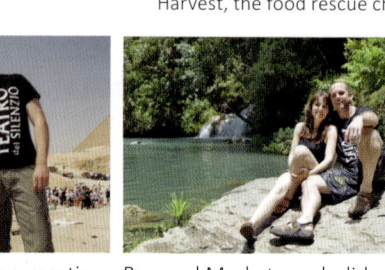
Ben and Marketa on holiday in Cuba.

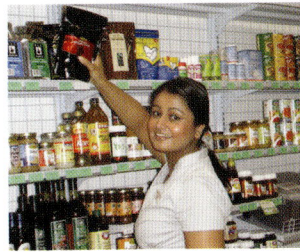
Ameeta in her health food store, Organic Matters, when it first opened.

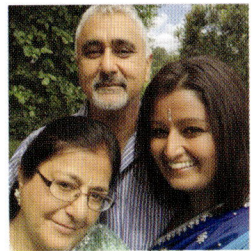
Ameeta all dressed for a function with her parents.

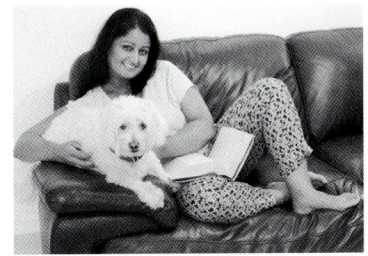
Ameeta Relaxing with a good book.

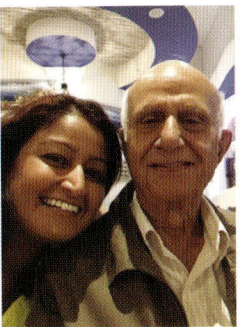
Ameeta and her grandfather having lunch in Johannesburg.

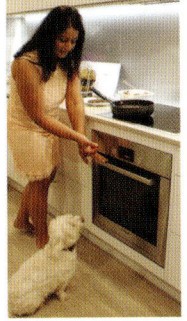
Ameeta spending time in the kitchen with her dog, Benji.

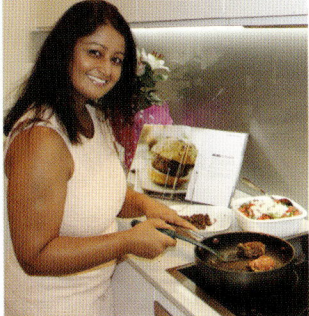
Ameeta cooking up a "healthy storm" for a dinner party.

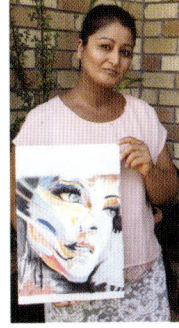
Ameeta with one of her recently completed art pieces.

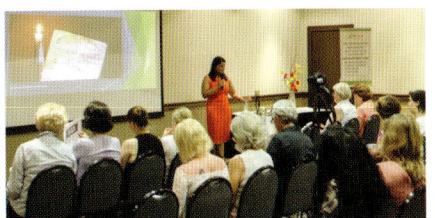
Ameeta Gangaram presenting at one of her events.

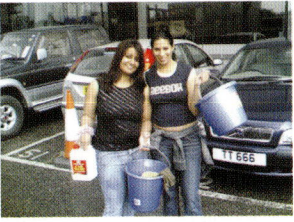
Ameeta Car Wash Appeal – London 2005.

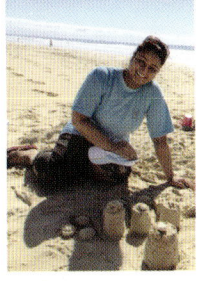
Ameeta Summerstrand beach relaxing 2015.

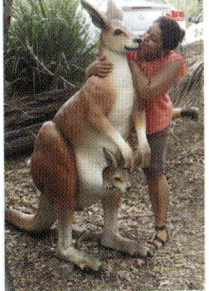
At Lone Pine Sanctuary having fun with the roo.

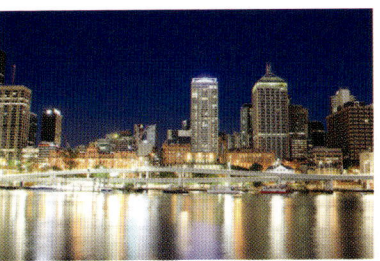
Ameeta's photo of Brisbane by night.

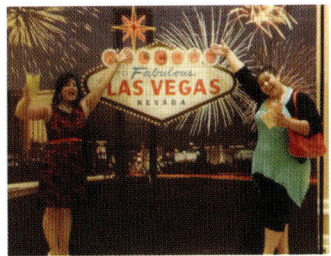
Having fun in Vegas.

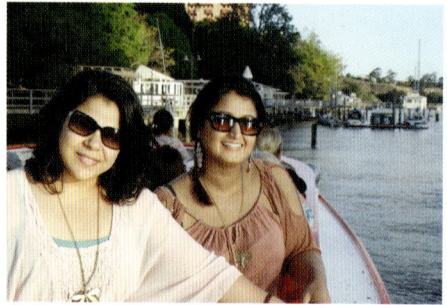

Having a timeout after first-ever Healthy, Happy Hormones event in Brisbane.

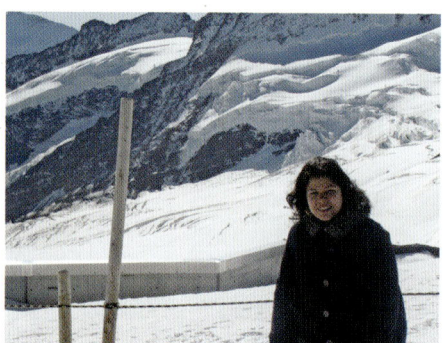

An adventurous trip alone to Jungfrau – Top of Europe.

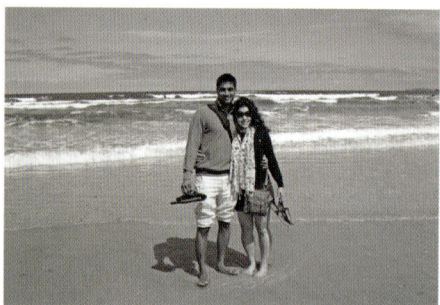

Shivi walking on the beach with her better half.

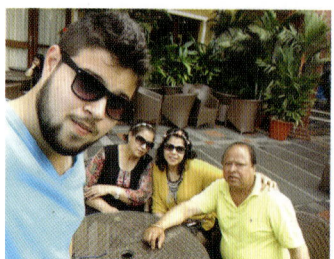

Chilling out with the family in Goa, India.

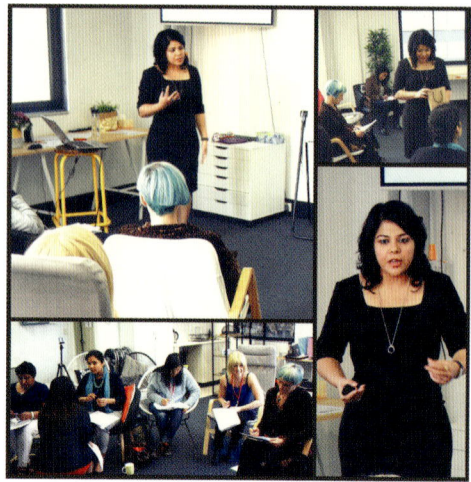

Shivi Chhabra sharing her message at the Healthy, Happy Hormones event in Sydney.

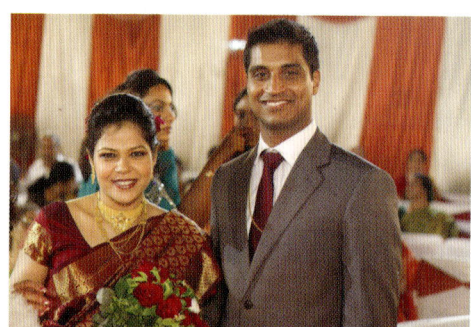

Part one: Shivi's big fat, Indian wedding.

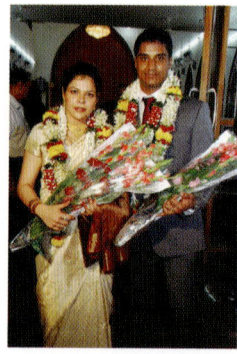

Part two: Shivi's big, fat Christian wedding.

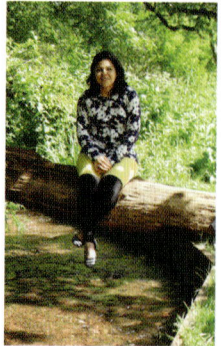

Walking through an unknown forest in Torquay, UK.

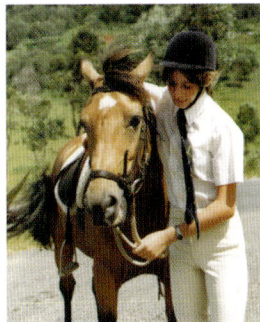

Heather and her "first love" horsing around..

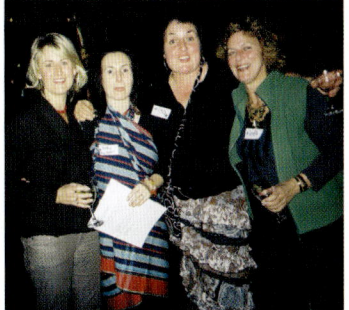

Charity fund raiser for the Hamlin Hospital Ethiopia with a big, beautiful bunch of heart-centred women.

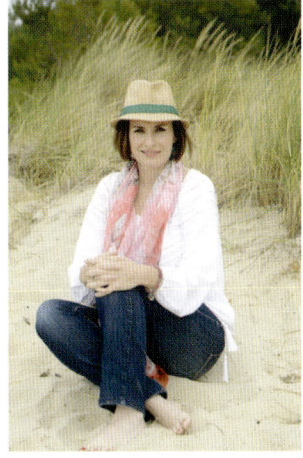

Heather Belle Murphy at the beach.

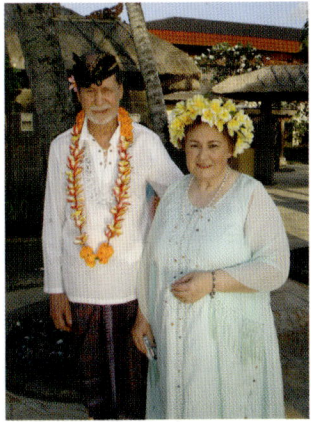

Heather's beautiful Mum and Dad in Bali.

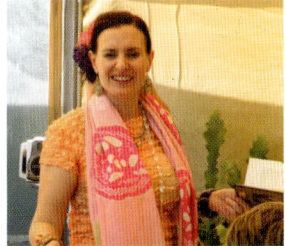

"Kahlil Gibram said what?!" Reciting The Prophet at a local arts event.

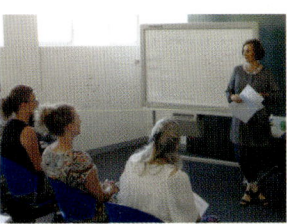

Sharing the love, living on purpose.

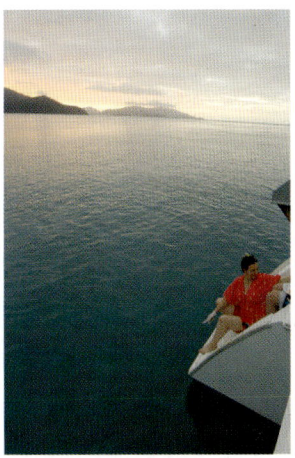

"Arrgh! It's a hard life at sea!" Cruising the Whitsundays.

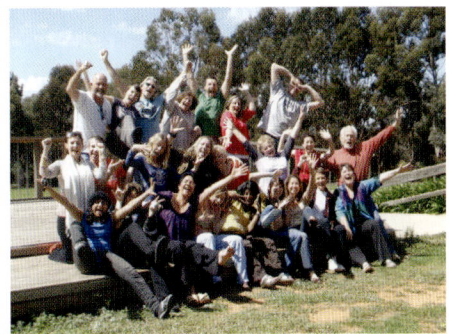

Heather making some noise with the Inner Peace Institute crew... just before the seven-day silence retreat.

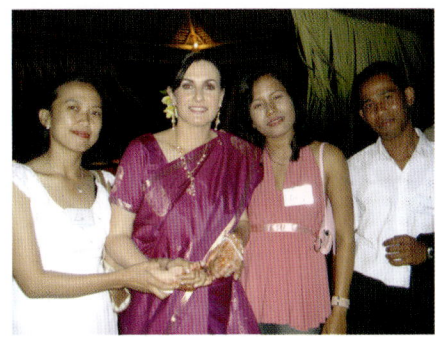

In Bali, one of Heather's favourite places, where people smile with their hearts.

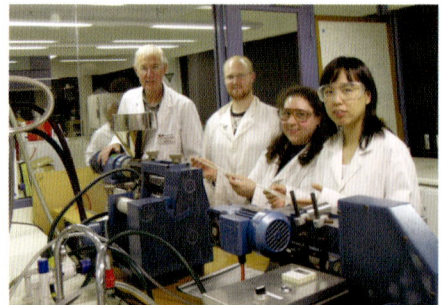

Research project team with Prof. Robert Shanks, Dr Kris Frost, Dr Antonietta Genovese and Dr Yulin Ji, creating biodegradable starch composite materials.

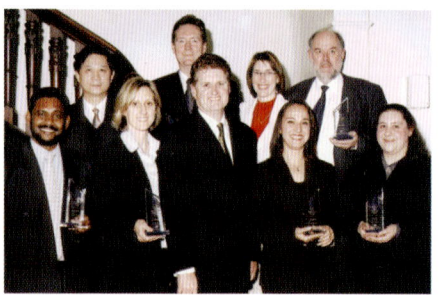

Research project team with Minister McGauran (2004) on development and innovation of passive fire protection composite materials.

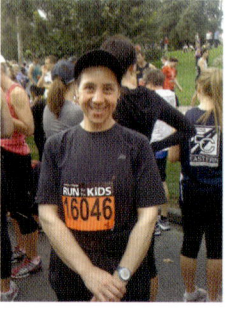

Antonietta at the starting line for the *Run for the Kids* fun run.

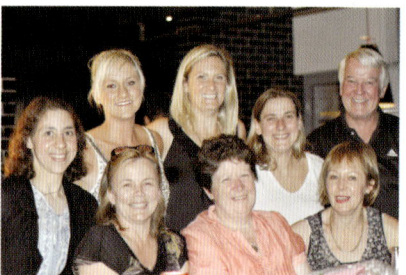

Celine and Antonietta at the local gym.

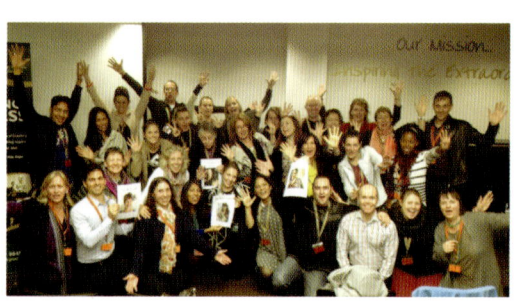

Vibrant community together celebrating the beginning a new journey of change at a foundations training.

Friday evening prior to the 14km fun run with fellow runners and friends.

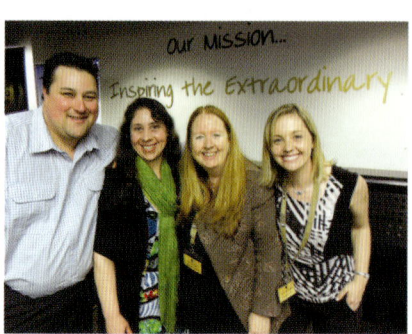

Luke, Antonietta, Mary and Tracy at workshop after presenting their talks.

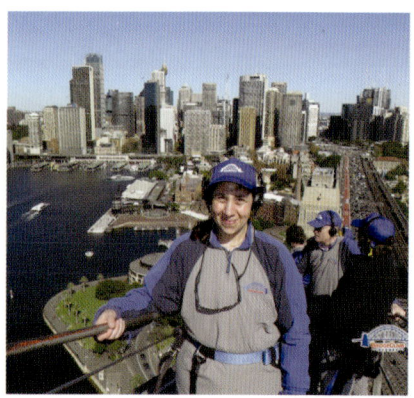

Leading the Sydney Harbour Bridge climb group. A picture-perfect day!

# Want to take the top 7 areas of your life to the next level?

*Start the 7 Day Transformation Today*

Simply go to www.elevate-books.com/you

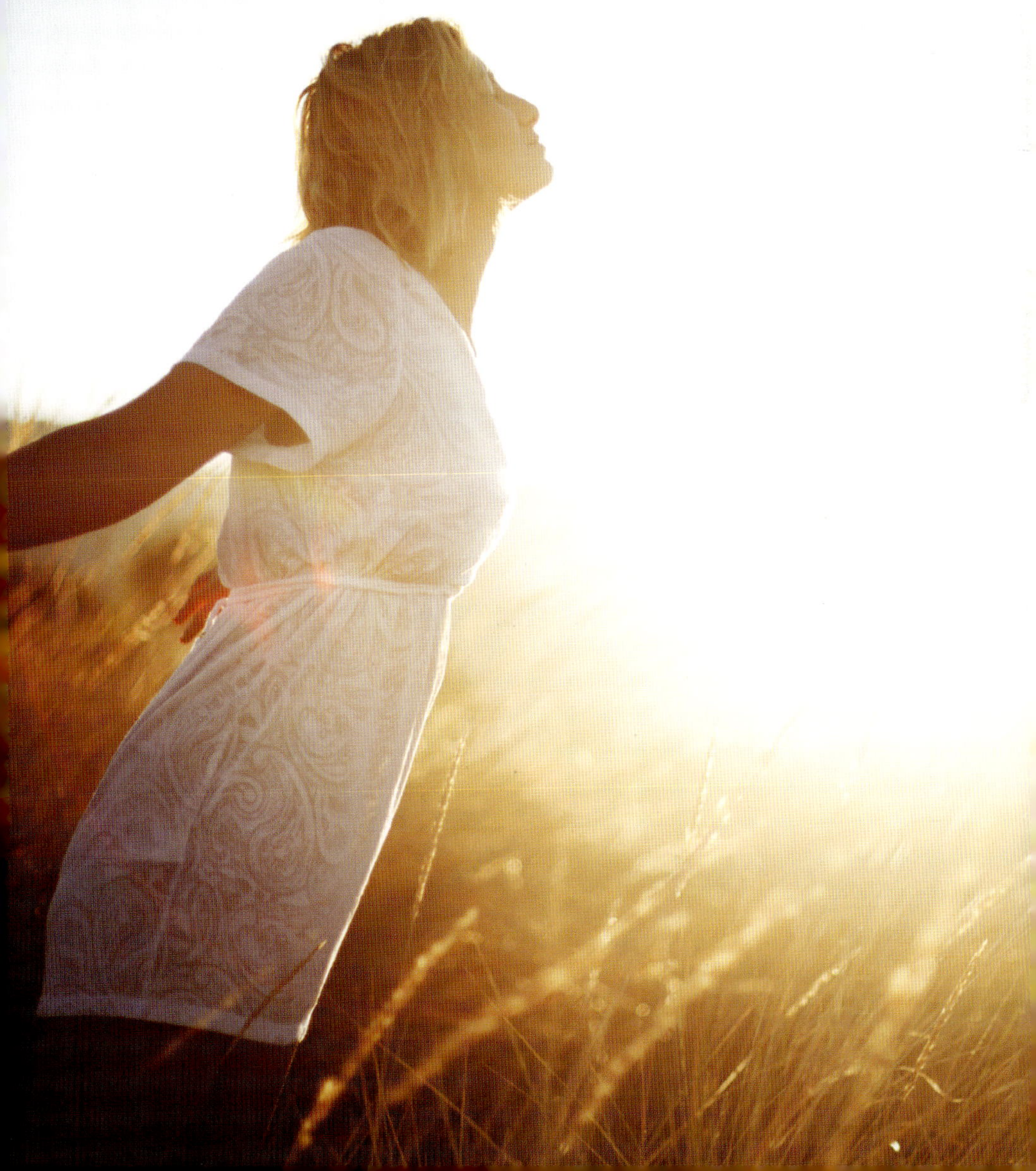

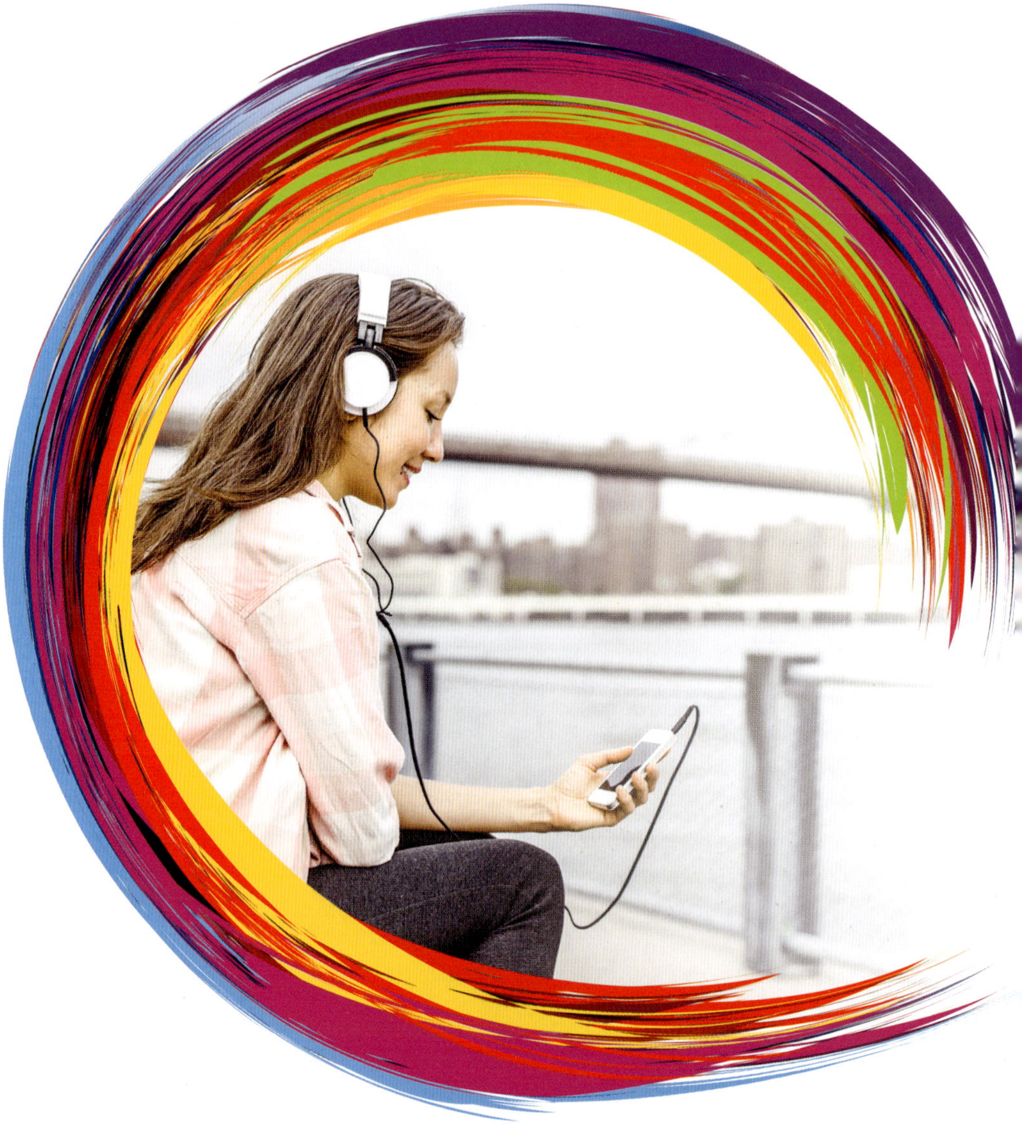

# Want to hear inspiring interviews from the authors?

*Listen to the elevate podcast.*

www.elevate-books.com/podcast

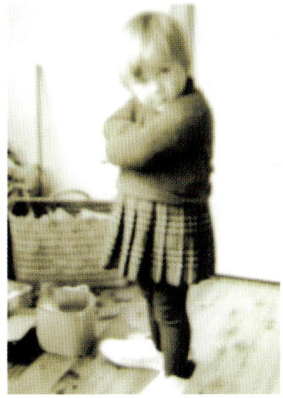

Libby displaying determination of spirit and fashion sense.

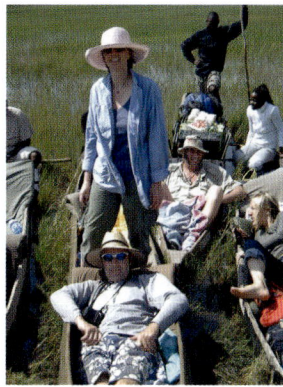

The mokoro, a gondola-type canoe, is the mode of transport around the Okavango Delta.

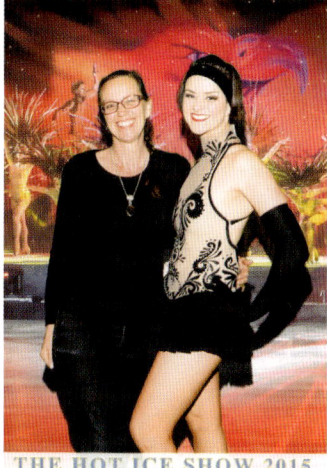

THE HOT ICE SHOW 2015

Libby Salmon with her daughter Elinor at Hot Ice. Photo courtesy of Redbox Photo Studio.

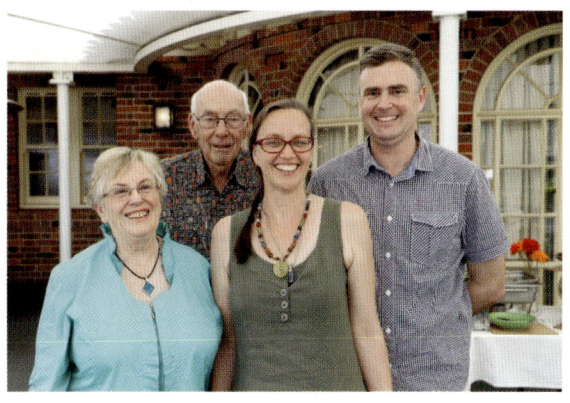

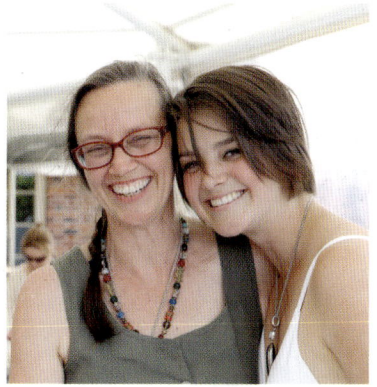

Libby celebrating her fiftieth birthday with her family.

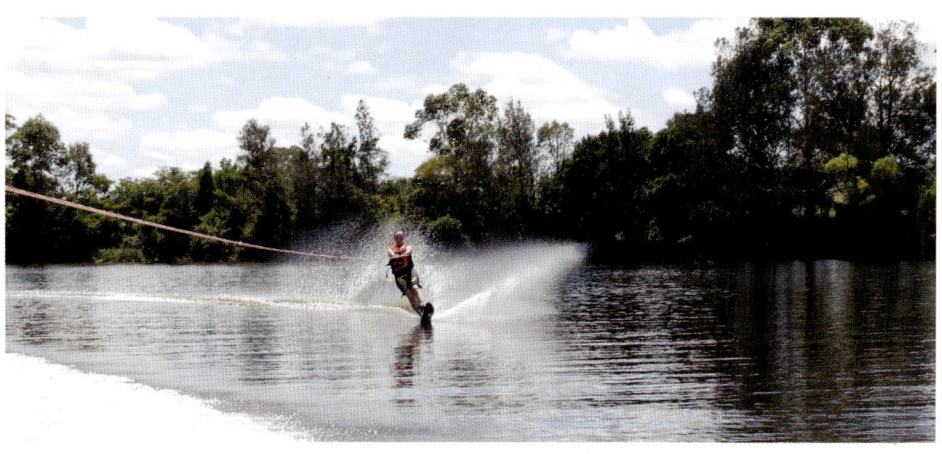

Libby waterskiing on the Williams River in NSW, a regular summer event.

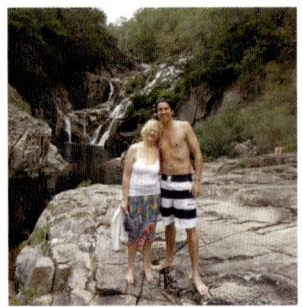

Engaging in one of Ruby's favourite pastimes, swimming in creeks near Cairns with her son, Alexander.

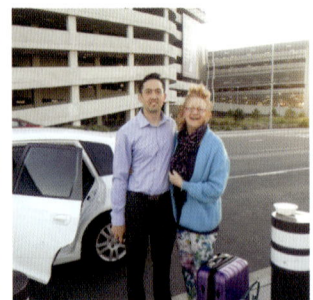

With son Matthew saying goodbye - a common theme in Ruby's life.

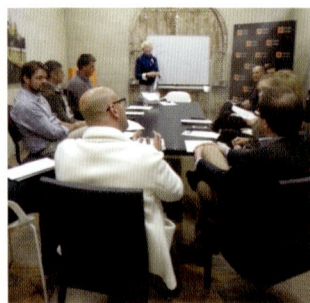

Ruby Johnson presenting to the Executive of Bird in Hand, an internationally acclaimed winery in the Adelaide Hills.

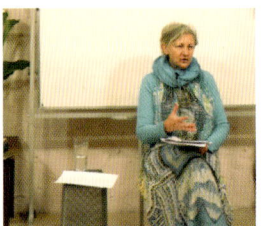

Ruby teaching her first Wholilstic Psychonomy class.

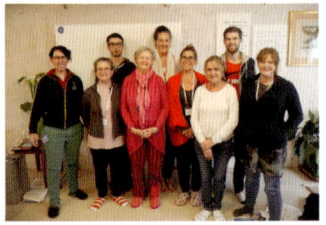

Ruby teaching Wholistic Psychonomy with a new group of trainees.

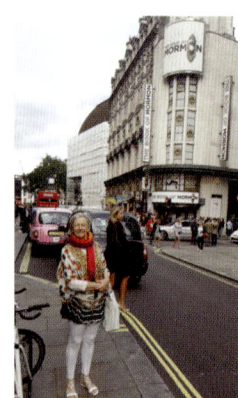

Ruby attending *The Book of Mormon.*

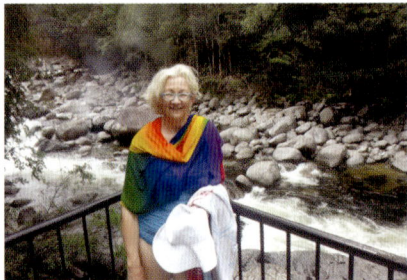

Ruby Johnson at the Rapids Crystal Cascades, Queensland.

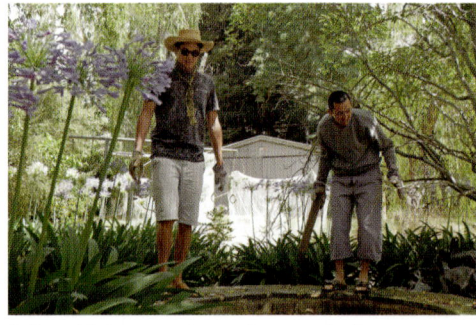

Ruby with her two favourite people, her sons, Matthew and Alexander, working in the backyard.

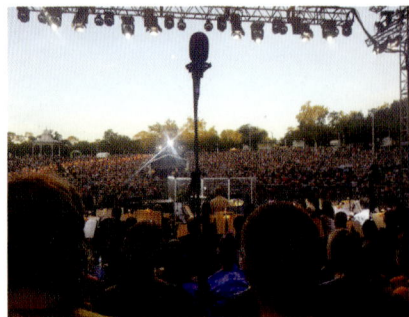

Ruby's view of Carols by Candlelight Christmas 2014 as a member of the Cantabile Choir.

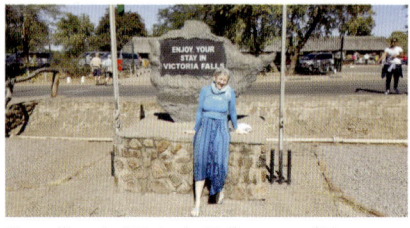

Travelling to Victoria Falls, one of the highlights of her journey to Africa.

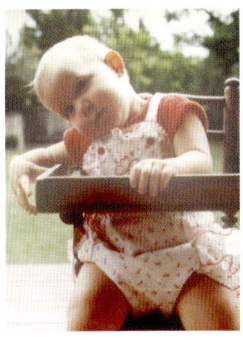

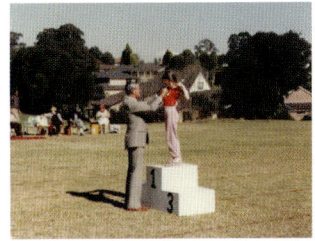

Jennifer's first win on the athletics track.

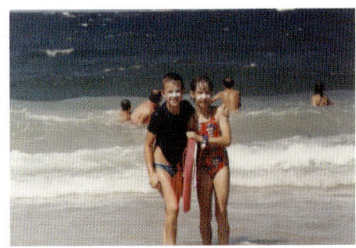

Fun in the sun and surf with her brother, Jason.

Just the beginning. So innocent.

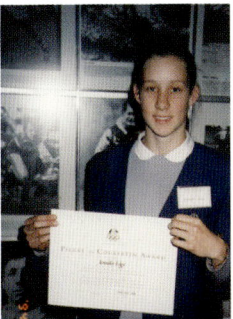

Jennifer receiving the Pierre de Coubertin Award.

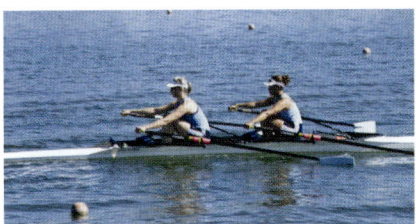

Competing at the Australian Rowing National Championships, 2012 (double scull with Laura Fau).

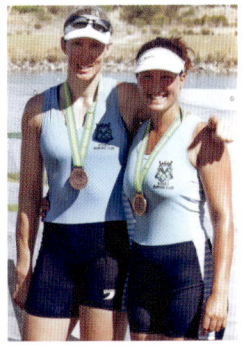

Bronze medal, Australian Rowing National Championships, 2012 (with Laura Fau).

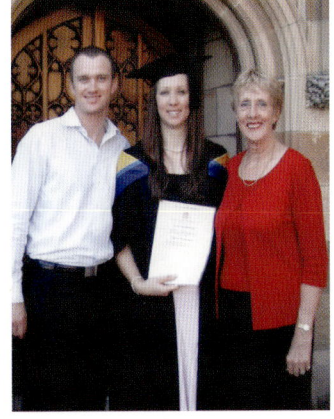

Jennifer Edge at her Masters of Physiotherapy Degree Graduation in 2004 (with her brother Jason and her mum).

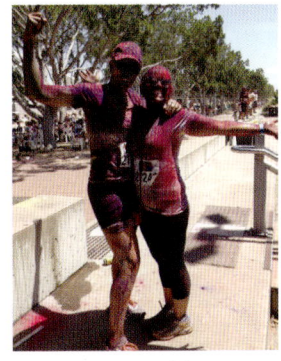

Getting messy raising money at The Color Run.

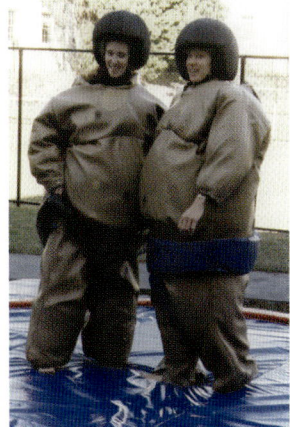

Sumo fun and laughter with her sister, Nathalie.

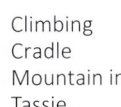

Climbing Cradle Mountain in Tassie.

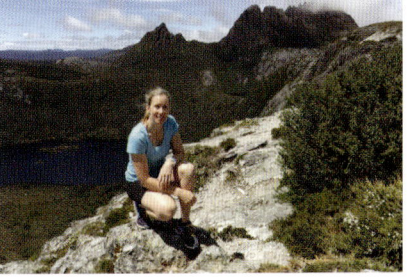

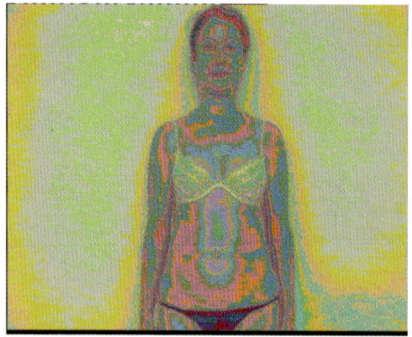

Catherine's Energy Scan.

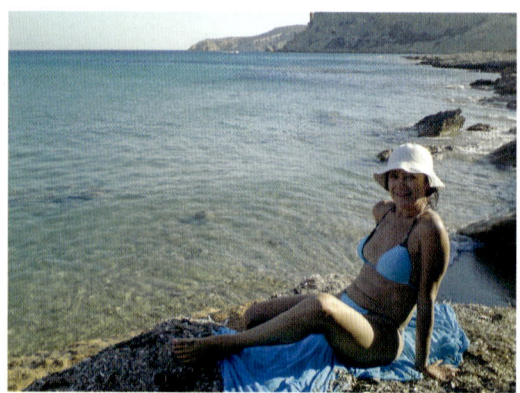

Catherine enjoying the healing waters of the Aegean.

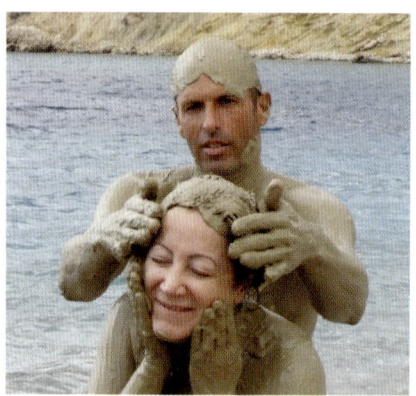

Catherine having a detox clay bath on the beach.

Catherine performing a crystal healing session.

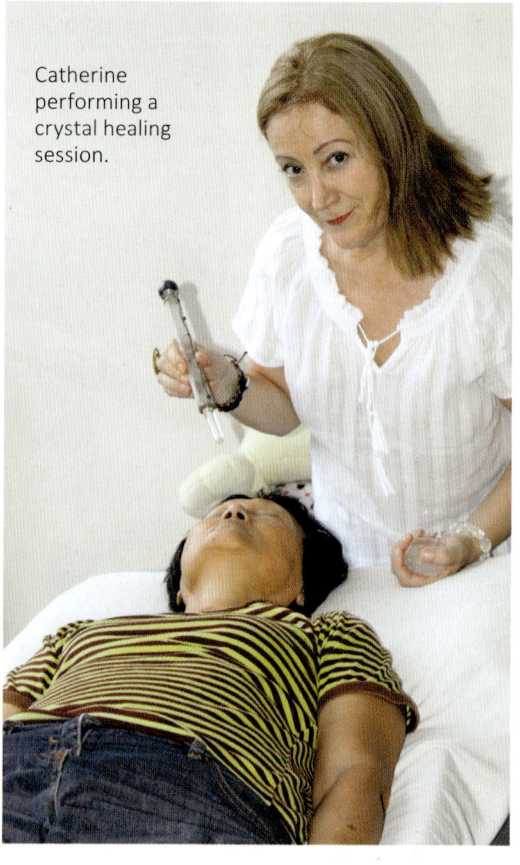

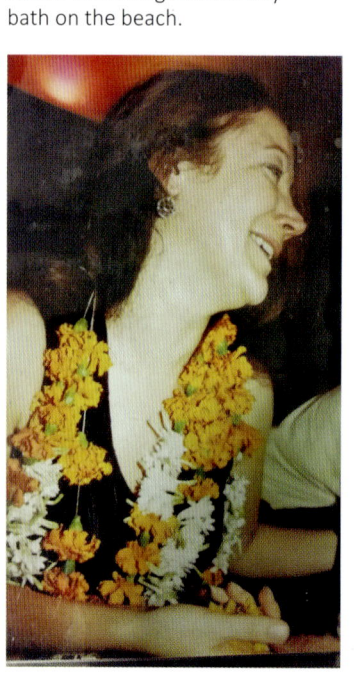

Catherine Printziou's Sannyas ceremony in India.

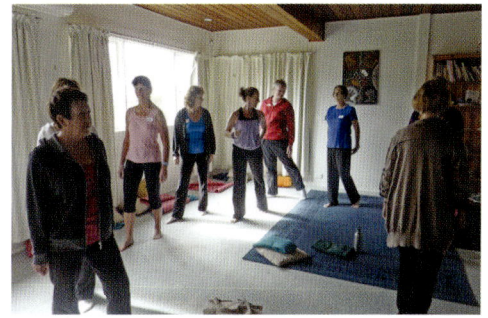

Maree Frawley inspiring muscular skeletal and emotional balance on retreat days.

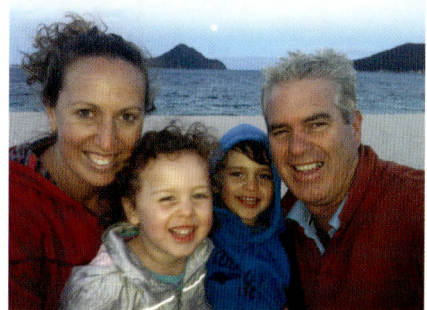

Maree, Kevin Katea and Kaiyu enjoying the sunset at Nelson Bay.

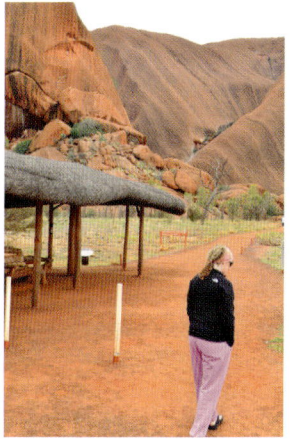

Enjoying reflection and the wonder of Uluru.

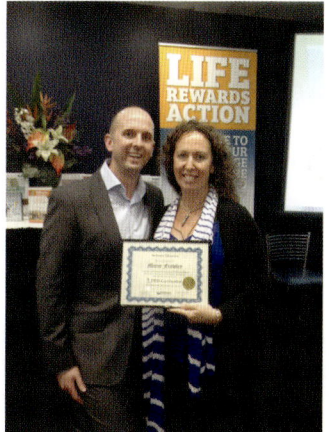

Maree with Ben Harvey at Authentic Education PHD graduation.

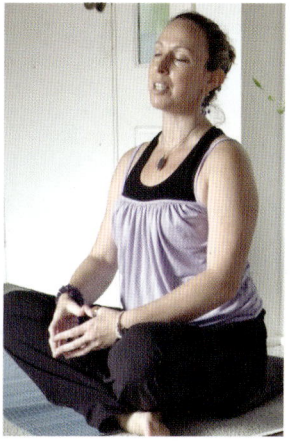

Maree practicing and instructing mindfulness through gentle yoga.

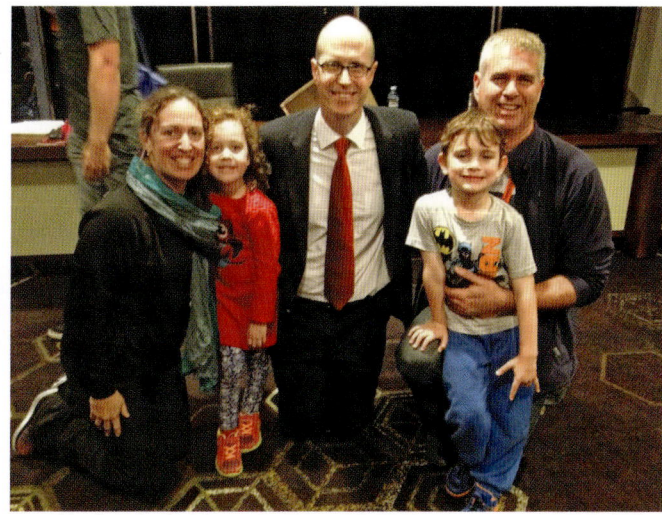

Maree, Kevin, Katea and Kaiyu with friend and mentor Steve McKnight.

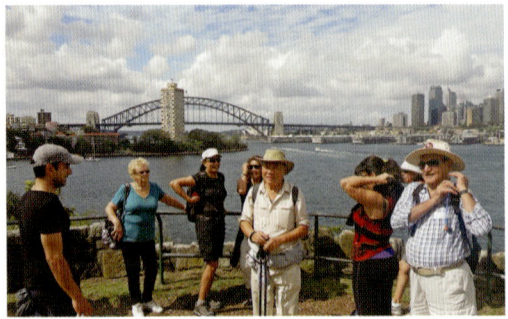

One of Russell's favourite pastimes: walking and talking.

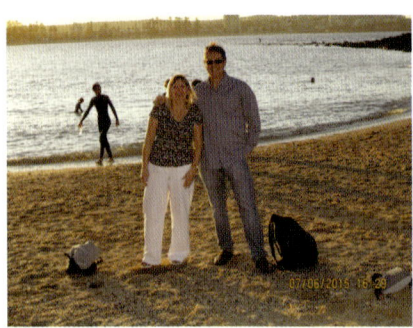

Russell with his sister, Heather Parker.

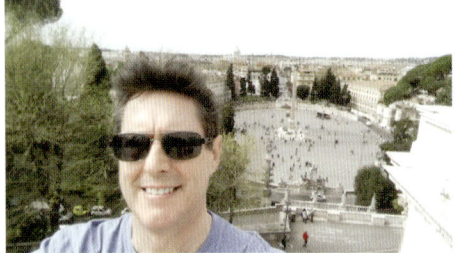

Russell in Rome's Piazza del Popolo, a majestic square in his most favourite city so far.

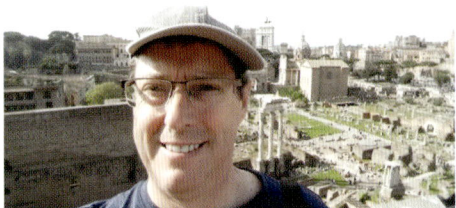

Russell taking the worst selfie in the best place – Rome.

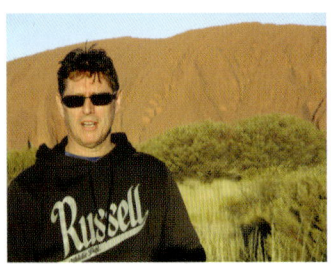

Russell, exhausted after driving four days to Uluru.

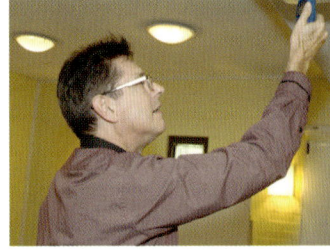

Russell Williams doing-a field survey.

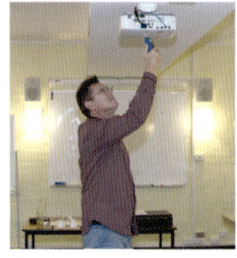

Russell measuring the electromagnetic field of a projector.

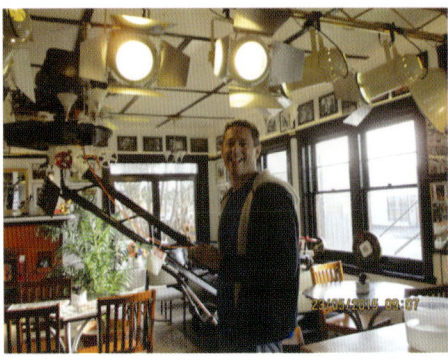

Russell star-struck in Tasmania.

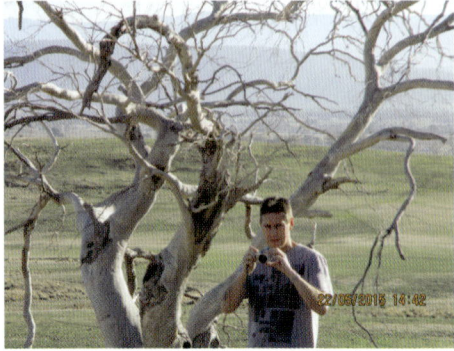

Russell on his road trip to Uluru.

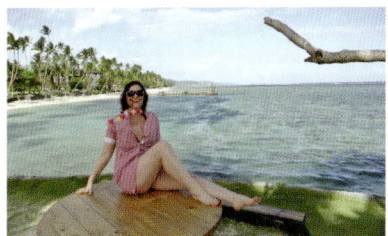

Suzy in Fiji in a school dress as part of her championship fundraising campaign for One Girl.

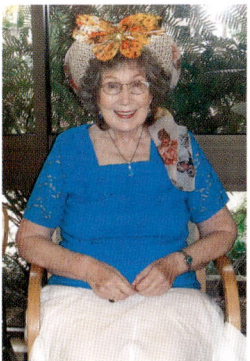

Suzy's mum, a woman with a heart of gold.

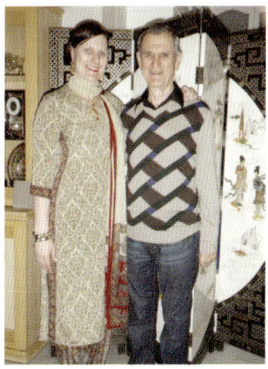

Suzy Jukes in a traditional Indian Sari in Pune with her dad.

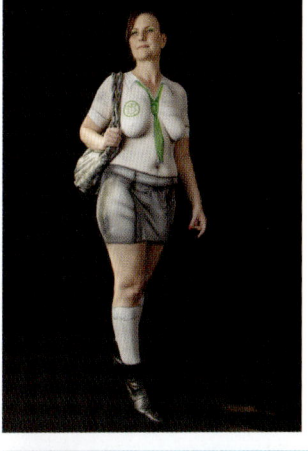

Baring all for charity: body painted in a school dress. (Artist: Gina Nomachi. Photographer: Colin Ellis)

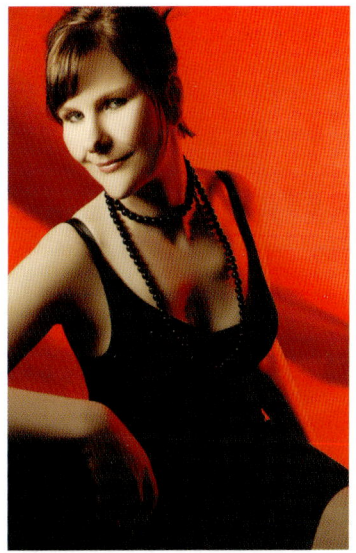

After winning $1100, Suzy got professional photos taken, which her mum always cherished.

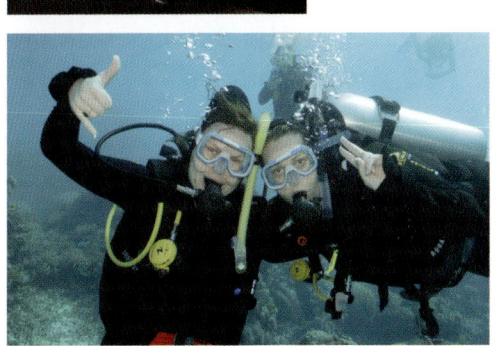

Suzy engaging in one of her passions, scuba diving.

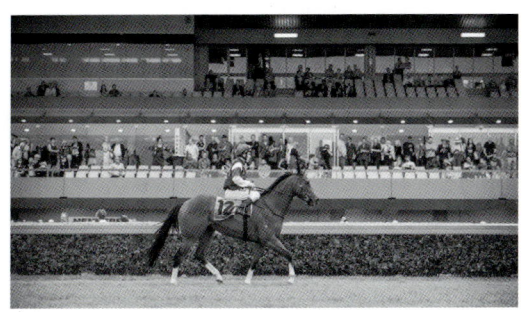

Suzy's champion race horse, Angelic light.

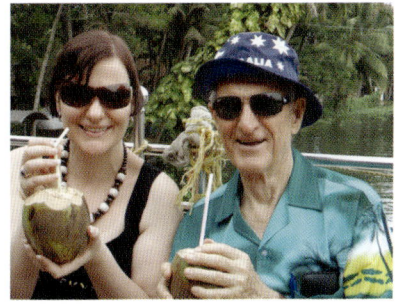

Suzy and her dad drinking coconuts on a houseboat in Kochi, India.

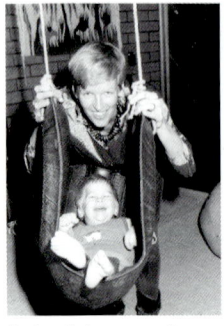

Anke doing exercises with her son, Friso, to help improve his brain function.

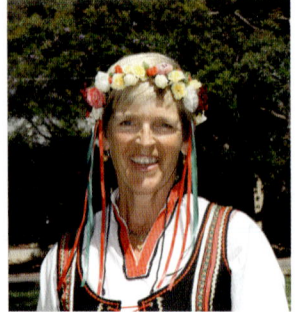

Anke in Romanian costume before a performance in a retirement home.

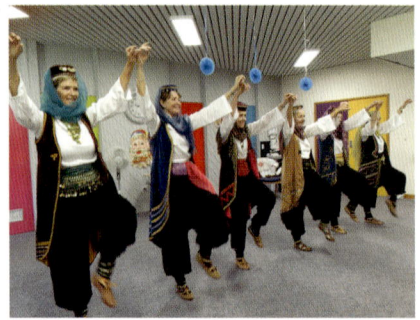

Živana performing a suite from Azerbaijan for Resthaven at their Christmas party.

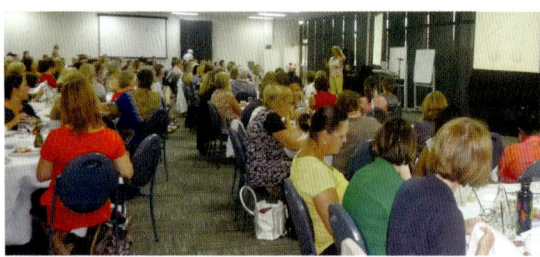

Anke Koelman training a large group of teachers and early childhood educators in "How to improve Autism and Autism Spectrum Disorders".

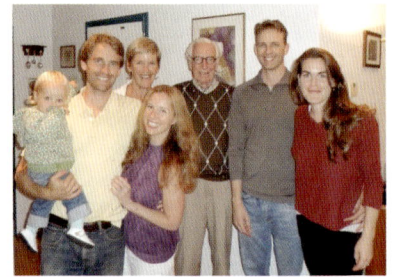

Family reunion in the Netherlands in 2015.

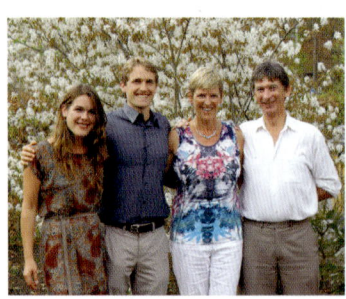

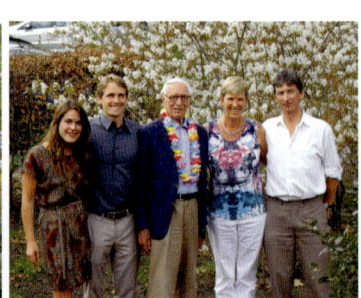

Family reunion in the Netherlands for her dad's eighty-fifth birthday.

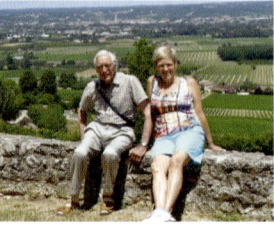

Anke meeting her first grandchild, Sasje, in the Netherlands.

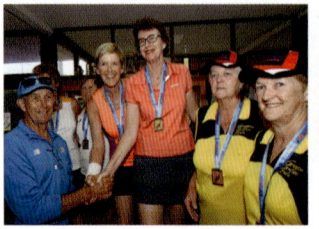

Anke and her partner, Debra Clarke, winning the gold at the Australian Masters Championships in 2015.

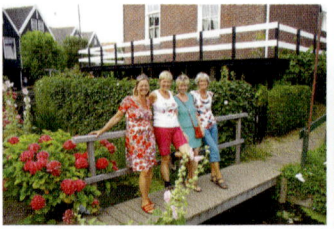

Anke and her sisters at the yearly Sisters Day in Marken, the Netherlands.

Anke on holidays with her dad in France.

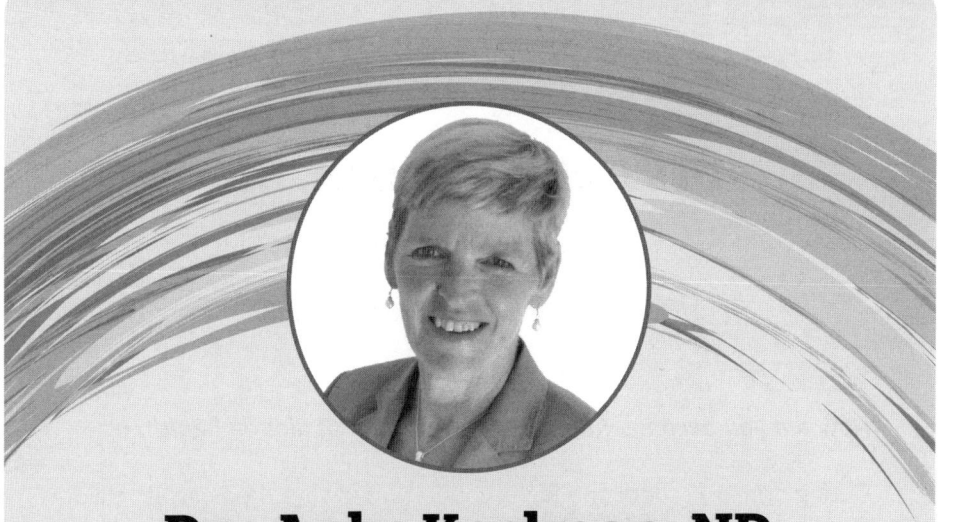

# Drs Anke Koelman, ND

## Gut Revelations

Anke Koelman was born in the Netherlands, where she graduated with a Doctorandus degree (Drs) from the University of Leyden in Biochemistry and Mathematics. She taught Organic Chemistry and Biochemistry at universities in the USA and UK before coming to Australia in 1984.

In 1985, her third child, Friso, was born with a severe brain injury. To help him improve, Anke learned many behavioural techniques such as kinesiology, Brain Gym® and Neuro-Organisation Technique. Friso also suffered from recurrent bronchitis, which led Anke on a journey that involved studying naturopathy, Western herbal medicine, homoeopathy and a Master's Degree in Health Sciences specialising in Nutrition Medicine and more recently the Biomedical approach to autism and chronic diseases.

Anke now specialises in autism spectrum disorders and other gut-related diseases and works in her private practice with children and adults. She also teaches professional development courses for teachers and early childhood educators.

# Drs Anke Koelman, ND

## Gut Revelations

### The Gut: The new frontier of health

*How did you become interested in the effect of diet on health?*

During primary school and high school I was always the heaviest child in the class, and I've counted calories since I was fourteen. I didn't eat more than other children, so I wanted to find out why I was overweight and others were not. If Nutrition Medicine had been available in 1971 I would have studied it, but since it wasn't I chose biochemistry instead and decided to become a teacher.

My mother was diagnosed with breast cancer in that year, and she investigated many diets that had been successful in fighting the disease. She decided to follow the Moerman Diet that had been successful in shrinking tumours in pigeons and followed it strictly for several years. I was sceptical at the time and thought that if the diet was so successful, every doctor would recommend it. However, despite the cancer coming back several times and in different places, she survived it for thirty-five years (later on with the help of nutritional supplements as well.) I became more curious and wondered how such a diet could have helped in beating a serious life-threatening disease.

In 1985 my third child, Friso, was born with a severe brain injury, which was later diagnosed as severe spastic quadriplegia. Because of the spasticity I couldn't breastfeed, and when he came home from the hospital I stopped expressing. This meant I had to give him baby formula, which was made from cow's milk. When Friso was a few months old, he had bronchitis that was treated with antibiotics. This seemed to cure it, but three weeks later he had bronchitis again. It became a monthly pattern: bronchitis, antibiotics, bronchitis, antibiotics, with no end in sight. He also became increasingly constipated.

Someone recommended a naturopath who said many children have problems digesting cow's milk and that due to the brain injury, Friso's body may not be able to drain his own lung fluid. The naturopath recommended a homoeopathic remedy called Pulmo-drain and said I should change to soymilk and take him off wheat products. It sounded a bit far out to my scientific mind, but I realised this pattern wasn't good for his health, so I decided to give it a go.

The bronchitis stopped, but three months later Friso started projectile vomiting, because he couldn't tolerate the soymilk either. The naturopath suggested changing to goat's milk, and that fixed it. He stopped vomiting, and he never had bronchitis again. I was amazed that one homoeopathic supplement and a simple diet change could have such a major impact on his body.

A few months later at one of his checkups, he was weighed and deemed too skinny, so the doctor made an appointment for him with a dietician in the children's hospital. She recommended whipped cream and custard to, in her words, beef him up. I was concerned, because that meant putting him back on cow's milk. When I mentioned his history of recurrent bronchitis, she dismissed any connection with cow's milk in no uncertain terms.

Reluctantly, I followed her advice, and ten days later Friso had his first-ever ear infection that was yet again treated with antibiotics. At the follow-up consult with the dietician, she dismissed this as a pure coincidence. I disagreed with her but said I would try one more time. Ten days later he had another ear infection and was treated with antibiotics again.

At the next appointment I asked to see the specialist instead. He said he'd heard there may be a connection between cow's milk and upper respiratory tract infections, so I took Friso off the cow's milk products, and he never had another ear infection.

It was clear to me that Friso's reaction to cow's milk was not a coincidence. I had non-stop ear infections myself until I was four years old, and my other son had them until he was two. Perhaps we were more sensitive to cow's milk than other people, so maybe it had something to do with our genes. If so, could other families be more sensitive to different foods in their diet?

This question intrigued me, and when the University of New England offered a Master's Degree in Nutrition Medicine for the first time in 2001, I immediately enrolled. The idea of using herbs to help the body heal also appealed to me, so I decided to become a naturopath, as well as a homeopath. I started attending international conferences where I learned about the latest developments in Nutrition Medicine, as well as two new sciences: Nutrigenomics, the study of how nutrients talk to genes and Epigenetics, the study of how the environment affects our genes.

I also discovered the link between cow's milk and ear infections, which is that cow's milk increases mucous production. Young children often have difficulty draining this mucous from their ears, and since mucous is a nice place for bacteria to colonise, this can lead to ear infections. It applies to upper respiratory infections as well.

### What are you passionate about?

I'm most passionate about the recovery of children with regressive autism. These children seem to develop normally at first. Then all of a sudden they stop communicating, lose interest in their surroundings and often make repetitious movements with their hands, known as stimming. Many times speech disappears, and children make squealing noises instead. Parents see their beloved child disappear in front of their eyes. These children are the canaries of our coalmine (our world).

**What has changed from the twentieth to twenty-first century?**

Acute infectious diseases have plagued mankind for centuries, and conquering them has been the main focus of western medicine in the last century. This resulted in the development of a large selection of antibiotics, anti-worm medications and an ever-increasing number of vaccinations.

At the same time, hygiene improved as most people in the developed countries gained access to tap water during the twentieth century and reduced the spread of Typhoid and Cholera. When flush toilets were invented and many homes were connected to a sewerage network, there was a further reduction. After the Second World War, nutrition also improved in many developed countries, which increased people's resilience to infectious diseases. Improved hygiene conditions also reduced the number of deaths during childbirth and early childhood, so by the end of the twentieth century people's life expectancy had improved in the developed countries. It looked like mankind had enriched its health by conquering infectious diseases.

However, at the end of the twentieth century the situation also changed for the worse in the industrialised countries. Childhood conditions such as allergies, eczema, asthma, childhood obesity, type I diabetes, attention deficit (hyperactivity) disorders (AD(H)D) and neuro-developmental conditions such as autism and autism spectrum disorders (ASD) were on the rise.

From 1987 to 2007, autism increased by fifteen-hundred percent, according to Dr. Kenneth Bock, M.D., author of *Healing the New Childhood Epidemics*. During this timeframe, the prevalence of chronic diseases such as obesity, cardiovascular disease, cancer, neurodegenerative and autoimmune diseases also increased.

An explanation may be found in changes that occurred at the end of the twentieth century:

▸ The amount of environmental toxins increased dramatically.

▸ The Western diet contained increasingly more processed foods that consisted of more calories, bad fats, added sugar and artificial colouring and flavouring, but fewer nutrients, less fibre and a reduced amount of fruits and vegetables compared to traditional diets.

▸ The invention of artificial preservatives made food preservation through fermentation superfluous.

At the same time there was an increased use of antibiotics and vaccinations, which had a profound effect on the health of the ecosystem in the intestines, also called the gut flora. The combined effect of these changes in diet, environment and gut flora reduced the resilience of many children and adults. The most vulnerable were those who'd inherited a genetic predisposition that made them less able to deal with these changes.

The sudden rise in ASD and the above-mentioned childhood conditions are a sign of the times. They are twenty-first century diseases caused by the world we now live in, to which many children have no adequate defences. The steep rise in chronic diseases shows that many adults are not coping all that well either.

### What organ is the most affected by these changes?

When I studied naturopathy, I was trained to look for a *Never Been Well Since* (NBWS) event when taking a patient's history, and I noticed that many symptoms seemed to start after a patient had taken antibiotics. These symptoms could be:

• skin rashes

• hay fever

- asthma

- food sensitivities and allergies

- irritable bowel

- weight gain

- fatigue

- thrush

- depression

- anxiety

- headaches and migraines

- joint pains

- sleeping problems

- mood changes

- thyroid problems

- type I diabetes

- recurrent infections

- regressive autism

Since antibiotics have the biggest effect on the gastrointestinal tract, often referred to as the gut, it seemed all of these diseases must have started in the gut, so I began studying it.

Pretty soon I discovered that in 400 B.C., Hippocrates, the reputed father of medicine, had already stated, "All disease begins in the gut". The question is: why and how?

### Can you tell me a little bit more about the gut?

The gut is a hollow tube that starts in the mouth and ends in the rectum. For all intents and purposes, what happens inside the gut happens on the outside of the body, and that's usually a good thing. The gut has many functions. Some are well known and others are not. Most people would know the gut helps to digest food, absorb nutrients into the bloodstream (on the other side of the gut wall) and eliminate undigested food particles from the body. It's less well known that the gut makes a number of vitamins and over seventy percent of neurotransmitters, such as serotonin, the feel-good molecule, and dopamine, which helps with motivation. This is why the gut is often referred to as a second brain.

The gut wall is a barrier that protects you from harmful microbes, toxins and undigested food particles that should not get into the bloodstream. It's covered with a thick lining, or biofilm, where many microbes live. Together they were often referred to as the gut flora, and more recently as the microbiome.

### How does the microbiome work?

The microbiome is an incredible ecosystem. When it's healthy, there's an enormous biodiversity of bacteria, fungi, parasites and other microbes that live happily in their own colonies, in harmony with the other colonies, as well as with their host, you. The human microbiome weighs around 2kg, and together the bacterial cells in the microbiome outnumber your human cells by ten to one. The bacteria fulfil a number of vital roles in your body. They make vitamins, help to digest food and play an important part in your immune function.

Babies are born with an immature gut and liver, which means they can't perform the functions an adult gut or liver can. This process of maturation can take up to six years.

Nature designed the human body in such a way that babies acquire their gut bacteria from the mother during the vaginal birth process and the breastfeeding period afterwards. Over the first year of life, whilst babies are still being breastfed, these bacteria learn to discriminate between self and non-self, as well as between beneficial and harmful microbes. This is called immune tolerance.

During this time, babies rely on the mother's antibodies to protect them from diseases, because they haven't reached the stage where they've developed immune tolerance, and they cannot make their own antibodies yet. This begs the question as to why most vaccines are administered during this particular period of the baby's development. It may also explain why most vaccinations need to be given three times, whereas if you have measles once at the age of four, you will have lifelong immunity.

**What happens when people take antibiotics?**

When you take antibiotics for a bacterial infection, the good bacteria that have learned immune tolerance in the first year of life, die along with the bad bacteria. This changes your microbiome and affects your immune tolerance. After taking antibiotics, many patients have said they became allergic to foods they'd never reacted to before.

When the good bacteria die, they leave an open space in the gut wall, which creates an opportunity for opportunistic fungi such as *Candida Albicans* to multiply. This can lead to thrush and/or brain fog. Depending upon the antibiotic that was used, some beneficial bacteria can survive as well. When they start to multiply, they too can become harmful. The microbiome resembles the ecosystem in a forest. If you shoot all of the owls, you may end up with a mouse plague. In the gut, a plague is usually called an overgrowth and results in a condition often referred to as *gut dysbiosis*.

Gut dysbiosis leads to gut inflammation and increased gut permeability, otherwise called *leaky gut*. The holes are big enough to let fungi, bacteria, toxins and undigested food particles through, which then enter the bloodstream and are transported to the liver where they need to be detoxified. If the liver can't eliminate these toxins, they can enter the bloodstream and be transported and deposited anywhere in the body. The immune system sees these particles as intruders that need to be attacked, thereby creating systemic inflammation, and this can result in any kind of *–itis* disease. The cause of many chronic diseases can be explained through this mechanism.

### How does diet affect the microbiome?

Your diet has an enormous effect on the microbiome and thus on your health. Some foods promote the growth of good bacteria that increase your health, while others promote the growth of "bad" bacteria, or fungi, that decrease your health. Here are some food facts:

▸ Sugar has a double negative effect on the microbiome. It stimulates the growth of *Candida Albicans* and is quickly fermented by bacteria, often resulting in bloating and gas.

▸ Wheat and dairy products are staple foods for many people in developed countries, but Professor Alessio Fassano, M.D. discovered that gluten from wheat causes a leaky gut. This means that after eating Weet-Bix, a sandwich or even just a piece of cake, toxins from the gut can leak into the bloodstream and into the brain where they can, and often do, interfere with brain function.

▸ Fermentation of foods is a great way to preserve them and obtain beneficial bacteria. These include sauerkraut, kim-chi and yoghurt. Artificial preservatives don't have the same beneficial effect.

▶ Fibre helps digestion and is beneficial to the gut bacteria. Most indigenous diets contain a lot of fibre, whereas processed foods contain little or no fibre.

I discovered that the Moerman diet that my mother followed after she was diagnosed with breast cancer, addressed all of these points. It excluded sugar, dairy and wheat and instead was high in vegetables and fibre, so it was ahead of its time.

The food you eat has an effect on the bacteria in your microbiome and recent research has shown that gut bacteria talk directly to your genes. If you eat junk food, your genes will respond by creating inflammation in your body.

### What has a positive or negative effect on the microbiome?

Stress has a negative effect on the microbiome, especially if this stress is chronic. Traumas such as a divorce or death of a loved one and unresolved traumas from the past can also affect the microbiome, and therefore your health, in a negative way.

A stressor is defined as something that causes stress to your body. Antibiotics, environmental toxins, a poor diet and poor lifestyle choices such as smoking, consuming large quantities of alcohol and a sedentary lifestyle are all stressors that have a negative effect on the health of your microbiome, whereas happy thoughts, exercise and a healthy diet have a positive effect.

### What's the solution?

Western medicine doesn't have a cure for chronic diseases, so prevention is the best approach. As the microbiome plays such an essential role in your health, it is important to focus on how to nurture your microbiome. When the microbiome is happy, the gut lining can heal, and when the gut is healthy, the chronic diseases will heal as well. Recently, Dr. Naviaux, from the USA, performed some interesting research studies with autistic mice and mice suffering from a chronic disease. His results showed that unless too much damage was done by the disease itself, most chronic diseases, including autism, were reversible.

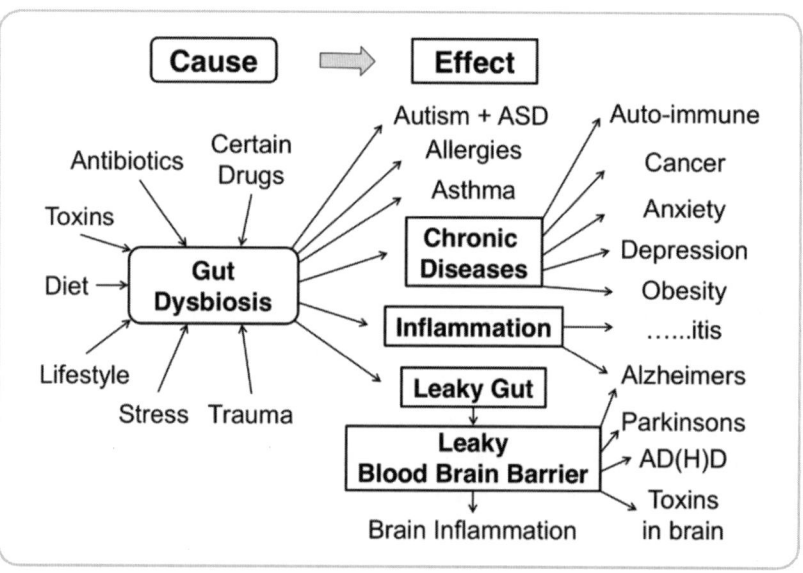

*Fig. 1 shows which stressors can cause gut dysbiosis and the effect this can have on the entire body.*

In another research study, when skinny rats were given a faecal transplant with the microbiome of obese rats, they became obese and vice versa, showing that the Microbiome plays a key role in what goes on in the rest of the body.

Your genes are important, but they merely determine your susceptibility to a disease. Your microbiome, together with diet, lifestyle choices, stress levels and the presence of environmental toxins, determines whether you will develop the disease or not.

### Can the Microbiome be restored?

Yes, fortunately it can. If you want to optimise your health, the ecosystem in the gut needs to be restored, and the leaky gut has to be healed and sealed.

The *RAPID* gut repair programme is a five-step process you can do to restore the microbiome and heal the gut lining:

▶ **R**emove all stressors to your gut

- Candida overgrowth

- foods that don't agree with you

- toxins

- excess alcohol

- stress and unresolved traumas

▶ **A**dd what's needed to heal

- nutrients

- digestive enzymes (proteins that help digest your food)

▶ **P**romote the growth of beneficial gut flora

- probiotics (friendly bacteria)

- prebiotics (promote the growth of healthy bacteria)

▶ **I**mprove the Immune system

- herbs

- essential oils

- nutritional supplements, such as zinc and vitamin C

▶ **D**etermine the best diet for your genes

Kinesiology is a great tool that can assist in determining what diet is best for you, what supplements your body may need and to find out what to remove from your diet, your environment and your body. You can find more information about kinesiology on the website www.optimumlearningandhealth.com.

### Can food have an effect on behaviour?

Many children with ADHD have had a reaction to one or more foods in their diet that interfered with their ability to concentrate.

A mother came to see me with her son who'd been diagnosed with ADHD. Kinesiology testing showed he was sensitive to wheat, so I designed a wheat-free diet for him. One week later, the principal of his school stopped the mother in the corridor and said, "Your son has been so well behaved this week, I take it you have finally put him on Ritalin (a drug often prescribed for children with ADHD)." The mother said: "No, all I've done is taken wheat out of his diet."

Since then, I've seen this many times with my patients. For children, as soon as the offending food is identified and removed from their diet, there's an immediate improvement in their development, learning and/or behaviour, and for adults it's their health and wellbeing.

I discovered that for me, the offending foods were sugar and dairy products, possibly as a result of years of endless antibiotics and an inherited sensitivity to dairy products. When I took them out of my diet, I lost 10 kg over a year without dieting and maintained this weight easily for thirty-five years.

**What determines when someone gets sick?**

Health is a function of two opposing factors: stressors and resilience. Resilience is your ability to cope with stressors. Imagine a bouncy castle. The people who are jumping on it are the stressors and the bouncy castle your resilience. When there are too many people for the strength of the castle, it will collapse (see fig.2).

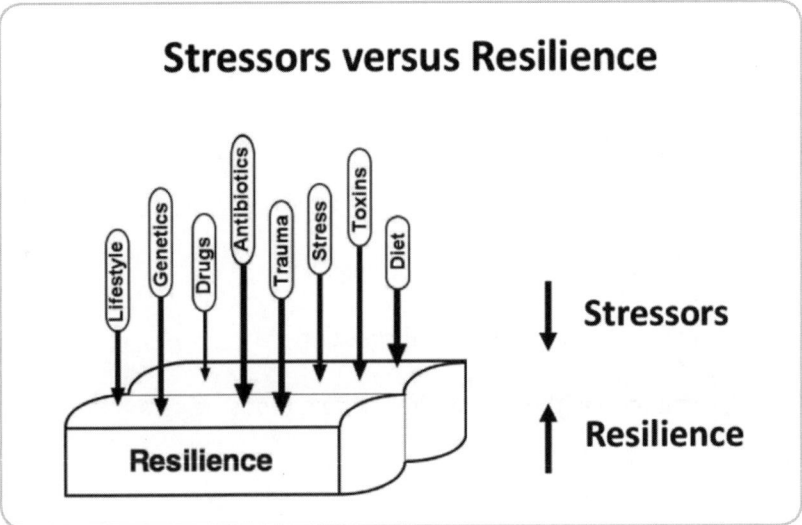

*Fig. 2 shows the two opposing forces that determine your state of health: the total amount and severity of the stressors and your resilience to cope with these stressors*

**How will a person know whether their gut is working properly? What signs and symptoms should they look out for?**

There are two kinds of signs and symptoms (S&S):

▸ the *obvious*

▸ the *not-so-obvious*

The obvious S&S are:

- bloating

- gas

- nausea

- heartburn

- bad breath

- bad body odour

- blood in the stool

- itchy nose or frequent sneezing

- extra mucous in mouth, throat or nose

- irritation in the throat after certain foods

- tummy pains

- smelly or loose stool

- constipation

- alternating diarrhoea and constipation

- undigested food particles in the stool

- hyperactivity or sleepiness after eating certain foods

The not-so-obvious S&S are the conditions and diseases that are the *result* of gut dysbiosis, such as:

- eczema

- sinusitis and rhinitis

- rashes

- hay fever

- asthma

- brain fog

- headaches and migraines

- fatigue

- irritability or mood swings

- depression

- anxiety

- ADHD

- autism spectrum disorders

- autoimmune diseases

- obesity

- obsessive compulsive disorders

- cancer

- Alzheimer's and Parkinson's Disease

- most chronic diseases

The best way to treat these conditions is to treat the root cause, which is the gut.

### Have you noticed any common denominators in children with regressive autism?

In my practice I've noticed that most of the children who regressed had received antibiotics before vaccinations, and the severity of their reaction to vaccinations had increased with every vaccination. Most of these children also had some genetic mutations that affected their ability to detoxify. Many had food sensitivities to staple foods, such as wheat and dairy products, and almost all children had gut inflammation, which in turn lead to leaky gut, brain inflammation and nutrient deficiencies.

### What's the most remarkable breakthrough you've seen in a child with regressive autism?

Adam came to see me when he was five and a half years old. He had no speech, squealed all day and walked aimlessly around the house, slamming his hand on tables and other surfaces. He didn't respond to his name and screamed if you tried to put him on his back. His bowels consisted of undigested food particles and smelled of the food he'd eaten. He was still wetting himself during the day and had white patches around his mouth, caused by Vitiligo and strange black patches on his arms and legs, which got him expelled from school. They were signs his immune system wasn't working properly.

Adam was the second of four boys, and for the first two years of his life he developed normally. He was generally a healthy boy, although during the first two years he suffered from many ear infections that were always treated with antibiotics. His vaccinations were up to date, and everything seemed fine.

When he turned two and seemingly without a trigger, he started to withdraw, stopped speaking and lost interest in his surroundings. Naturally, his parents were concerned and wondered what was happening to their child. As time went by, he became worse, not better. He received speech and occupational therapy, but nothing seemed to help. Eventually he was diagnosed with regressive autism, for which there is no known cure. His future looked very bleak.

When Adam came to see me, I knew this was a complex case that would need an integrated approach of many therapies. I started with the RAPID gut repair programme and used homoeopathic remedies and herbs to support his organs and immune system.

His bowels normalised within four months, but most of the symptoms persisted. After seven months of treatment, it seemed that we'd hit a brick wall. I decided I needed to investigate further and organised some functional pathology and DNA tests. They revealed Adam had *pyroluria*, which means an increased need for Vitamin B6 and Zinc. He also had a number of gene mutations in important metabolic and detoxification pathways. On the basis of these test results, I made up a new mix of vitamins and minerals and added a mixture of powerful antioxidants to the list of supplements in order to lower the inflammation and help with the detoxification processes.

Two weeks later I saw him again, and something had obviously changed. He sang "Old MacDonald had a farm" and was babbling. He also responded to his name and looked me straight in the eyes. I was impressed. All of that after one additional supplement.

He now wanted to be with his parents and play with his brothers. If something fell off the table, he would pick it up. His squealing had decreased substantially and he slammed his hand a lot less. His father said the new behaviours came and went, which told me that toxins and/or lack of nutrients could be responsible.

For the first time, Adam indicated he needed to go to the toilet during the consultation, and whilst we discussed his supplements, he walked over, put his arm around me and caressed my arm while smiling at me. I was so moved. It felt like we'd made contact on a soul level. This was the most inspiring moment of my entire professional life. He still had a long way to go, but the door to recovery had finally opened.

### Do you have any other inspiring stories?

In 1992 I was invited by the Zonta club in Haarlem, in the Netherlands, to hold a talk about kinesiology. There was a mix-up about the dates, so when I arrived no one was expecting me, because that night was dedicated to welcoming a new member named Nancy. At the end of my talk, Nancy asked what kinesiology could do for chronic fatigue syndrome (CFS). She'd been suffering from it for nine years (which started after she had food poisoning whilst overseas), and had seen many doctors, but there was no significant improvement.

Nancy came to see me the next morning. She brought along twenty-two pills that had been recommended by a naturopath, which she took every day. She told me that for many years she'd stay in bed twenty-two out of twenty-four hours a day. Though she'd improved slightly over time, she had to spend the whole day in bed just to be able to attend the Zonta meeting. She had a three cm ringworm patch on her cheek that wouldn't go away, because her immune system wasn't working properly. She was twenty-eight years old, married but had no children. She didn't study or work, because she was too tired to do anything.

What caused it all to go so wrong for Nancy at such a young age? Through kinesiology testing, I was able to identify the main, unresolved traumas that were causal to her CFS. The food poisoning that followed these traumas was merely the straw that broke the camel's back. Her adrenals were exhausted from dealing with the long-term chronic stress from the unresolved traumas, and she developed CFS.

Nancy had four sessions with me over the next three weeks. During those sessions, I used kinesiology to deal with the unresolved traumas and did an integration process for her immune system. This turned on systems in her body that had been switched off for years, such as her immune and digestive system. Through kinesiology testing I also determined which foods were beneficial for her and which ones were not.

The results were striking. Only one month later she was able to work fulltime, and she started catching up with nine years of living she'd missed out on. A year later I saw her again, and she said she was doing great but had trouble getting pregnant. This was not surprising, as her lifestyle of making up for lost time during the last year hadn't been conducive to getting pregnant. She had another kinesiology session, and within three months she fell pregnant and gave birth to a beautiful, healthy daughter. She subsequently had two more children. I never saw her again, but fifteen years later I became curious to know how she was doing, so I contacted her. She replied by letter, and you can find it in the *testimonial* section of my website at www.optimumlearningandhealth.com.

### What's the best thing that's ever happened to you and why?

The best thing that ever happened to me started out as the worst, which was the birth of my second son, Friso, who was born with a severe brain injury. It changed my life completely.

Through my journey with Friso, I learned many skills that helped improve his brain function and overall health. Sadly Friso passed away shortly before his eight birthday, but I decided to stay on the path I was on and become a health practitioner and trainer. Since then I have shared what I've learned over the last thirty years with many teachers and parents and assisted children and adults from all over the world with their journey towards health.

I remained in Adelaide and I was fortunate enough to meet my wonderful husband, Stewart, in 2003 while on a bus travelling from Canberra to Adelaide after teaching folk dancing, another one of my passions, at the National Folk Festival.

### What's your biggest life lesson?

Go with the flow of life, accept what life deals you and make the best of it.

### What's your simple formula for health?

Decrease the amount of stressors in your life and improve your resilience.

### How can someone best transform their health?

The best way to transform your health is by following the *ADORE* life process.

▸ **A**wareness

Start listening to the signals your body is giving you. The earlier you notice a symptom, the more you can do about it. When diagnosed with a disease, most people will say they didn't perceive any warning signals, but when asked to pay attention to the details, they can often identify that everything wasn't a hundred percent for a while prior to diagnosis. The best medicine is preventative medicine.

▸ **D**iet

Determine the diet that's best for your genes and your microbiome. Identify and remove the foods that are stressors to your body. You can identify these foods by functional pathology testing, kinesiology testing and/or paying attention to the way your body responds to the foods you eat.

Beware of food cravings, as the compulsion to eat these foods may come directly from the microbes that need that food to survive and thrive. Candida and some "bad" bacteria need sugar for their survival, so next time you crave a piece of cake, bread, pasta or pizza, ask yourself: *Who am I serving here?*

If you want to make a start towards finding out what your optimal diet is, determine which foods in your diet contain gluten and dairy, then do a hundred percent gluten and dairy-free trial for six weeks and see how you feel.

▶ **O**bserve

Notice what thoughts, emotions, memories, people or activities are causing a stress response in your body and where in your body you feel this stress. Some people feel it in their shoulders, whilst others feel it in their stomach, clench their jaw, or grind their teeth at night. Give the intensity of the feeling a number between one and ten, so you can start to monitor your stress responses.

▶ **R**emove

Eliminate as many stressors from your life as possible. This may mean a change in diet, job, partner, lifestyle, environment or attitude, such as the way you look at a situation. In my experience, a feeling of *No Choice* or *No Control* has the most profound effect on health. Kinesiology can help you to identify and deal with your stressors.

▶ **E**nhance

Improve your resilience by eating the foods that are right for you and your microbiome. Have a good work and play balance, sleep well, smell the roses, do what you love, enjoy life, and be with the people and/or animals you love.

In other words, become your own private health detective, because you're the only person who's present all of the time.

Good health may well be the most precious asset you will ever own. It's easier to maintain than to regain your health, so develop a proactive attitude. This means you need to listen to your body and attend promptly to the little issues like rashes, headaches, fatigue, gut symptoms, weight gain or stress, in order to avoid the big issues later on.

### What's the biggest tip you could give people?

Look after your gut, and your gut will look after you. Following antibiotics or certain drugs, do the RAPID gut repair programme to restore your microbiome, heal your gut lining and prevent long-term ill effects on your health.

### What's your best success tip?

Follow your heart, set a goal and achieve it.

 To discover more about how Anke can help you *Elevate Your Health*, visit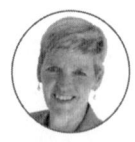

www.elevate-books.com/health

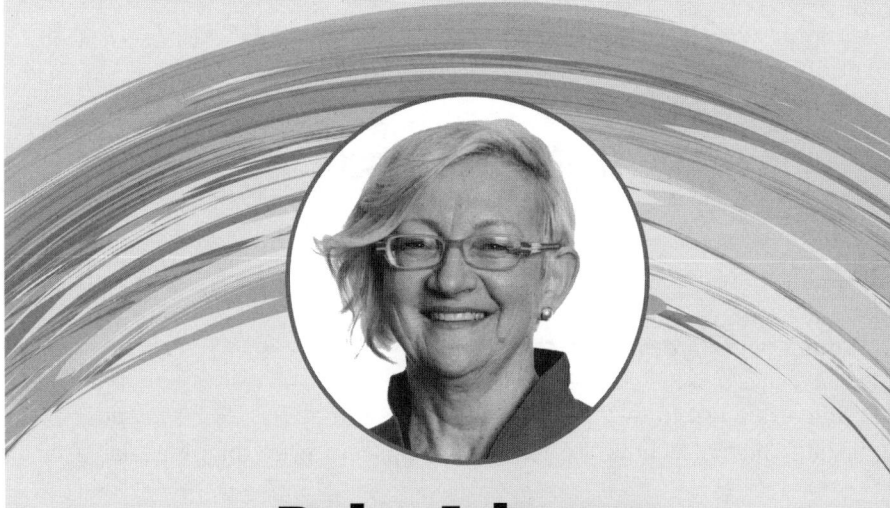

# Ruby Johnson

## Beat the Binge

Ruby is an experienced coach of over twenty-five years. She specialises in Wholistic Psychonomy, which studies the laws of the personality and the soul.

She's the author of three books on the topics of emotional and mental wellbeing, coping with the effects of addiction and re-empowerment after sexual assault.

Ruby holds an Honours Degree in Psychology, a Diploma in Education and a Bachelor of Education.

She's been to hell and back, both personally, and professionally, and has made it her mission to help anyone in need, from all walks of life. As a result, she's worked with everyone, from an outlaw motor bike gang president, drug addicts and prostitutes, to professionals, corporate executives and business owners.

Ruby digs deep to find her clients' true desires and is passionate about getting real results.

# Ruby Johnson

## Beat the Binge

### What's your biggest life lesson?

I've learned not to take life too seriously and that *This, too, shall pass*, because no matter how dire a situation may seem, everything is healable.

I learned this lesson the hard way when I was thirteen and my sister, who was twenty at the time, was murdered. She had a kid who was two years old named Alwyn, and after her murder my parents adopted him, which made him my brother. Then my parents were killed in a light aircraft crash when I was nineteen, so that meant by the time he was nine he'd had had four sets of parents. That's a lot to handle for anyone, let alone a child.

### What inspired you to be a coach?

Seeing my older son lying curled up, sobbing about how worthless he was. At that time he shared with me a life event he'd been carrying around for the five preceding years. This incident only surfaced after he'd given up smoking dope. That he knew the source of his pain and carried it for so long before sharing it with anyone, still really gets me. This was one of the reasons I was driven to start the *Beat the Binge* program.

It became a turning point for me. Nothing prepared me for seeing my son like that. There was so much pain and shame. Following this event, he went to an AA meeting where he realised there were other people like him. Unfortunately, like many others, AA didn't suit him, and he only went twice. Over the next couple of years he began to turn his entire life around. It wasn't smooth sailing, but he evened out. Now he's happily married, and life is really working well for him.

What also inspired me to be of service to others is understanding that most people deal with grief and difficult memories the way I did. The night of my parents' funeral, I bayed at the moon and metaphorically pulled down a shutter between me and the deep wound I experienced as a result of their deaths. I didn't let it affect me for fifteen years, or so I thought, and just got on with my life.

Part of the process I help people with is that gradual working through and transforming of their lives, so those memories no longer drive them.

I think I got through my traumas because I had resilient parents. They were reading books about isometric exercises and the *Kama Sutra* when I wasn't even a teenager. They never talked that much about it. I found the books after their death. I think I was fortunate my parents didn't have a traditional approach. This was in the early fifties, so it was way before these concepts became popular in the sixties and seventies.

Having that as part of my conditioning and the attitude of, *You just have to get on with it,* really helped me. My father used to say, "Well, honey, if you can't laugh at yourself, who else is there?" By the age of thirty-two, I regarded my life as a total mess. I looked good on the outside. I had my husband and two children, along with the house, the car and all of the trappings, but on the inside, over those fifteen years when I wasn't consciously dealing with my parents' death, I just shut off my feelings. I'd stay up designing dresses and sewing until three in the morning. I was teaching all day and had two kids to take care of. Then my marriage broke up, and I became a single mum.

Eventually I got to a place where I knew I had to do something. The real turning point in my life overall was seeing the word *rebirthing*, a form of therapy involving conscious, connected breathing that often triggers the trauma of being born. I had no clue at the time about the specifics, I just knew it's what I needed. I arranged a session with someone, and it quickly became evident she had no real training in that area. After the "session" I said to my then partner, "If that's rebirthing, I don't want to have anything to do with it. But I know it's not, so I'll keep looking."

I found somebody who later became my teacher. We had this breath session that literally changed my life. I had such a bad back at the time that I couldn't sit in a normal chair or drive a car for longer than five to ten minutes at a time. After this one breath session, this amazing light went right where I had the troubled spine. I had a revelatory experience.

At the end of the session I sat with my legs crossed, which I hadn't done for years. Then I drove forty minutes straight home, without realising I was doing it. In fact, it took me about six weeks to comprehend what an impact this one session had had on my life. Have you ever noticed how you can undergo incredible experiences, and all of the changes that result from it only become evident in bits and pieces after the event? This session was so powerful that I decided to train as a rebirther and to this day I use breathwork as one of my major tools.

What took me down the path of getting into coaching and helping people change their lives was not only doing the rebirthing training but also all these other new-age, hippie, far-out methods, including crystal healing. As a result, I wanted to assist others in having the same kind of transformation I'd had.

Because of what happened with me, I knew what was possible. As a result, I do my best to act as a guide to create similarly powerful changes for others. Everyone needs to go through the various stages of life: baby, toddler, child, teeny, young adult, and eventually, adult. In my experience, nobody, no matter how brilliant you are, can miss out on any of these stages. I don't mean on just the physical plane but the emotional, mental and spiritual as well. I wanted to help people ascertain what stage they were at without making it wrong, find out where they wanted to go and help them get there. I set up a practice and created groups and then trainings. I just didn't think I could fail, and I didn't.

**Is there one story of transformation that really stands out for you?**

Recently, I had a couple come and see me. The man had been diagnosed with terminal cancer. He was no longer concerned about himself, because he'd come to terms with his condition. His wife had a problem with alcohol and refused to admit she had one, which in itself is a common problem. She had five children to take care of, and that's a lot to manage alone.

At the end of that first conversation the husband also decided to see me, so we set up a long-term program where one of them would come one week and the other would come the next. The husband had been told he had less than a year to live. We started working together in March, and by October he was in total remission.

I think that's a pretty remarkable outcome. In addition, the wife went from saying, "No, I don't have a problem, but I know it's a problem for him, so I'll come along, even though nothing ever works for me" to three months later realising she did have a problem. Once she understood it was impacting her relationship, we could go through all of the steps, which I teach in my five-week *Beat the Binge* program. Now they're both leading much happier and healthier lives.

**What would you like your legacy to be?**

For me, a legacy is not about who I am or what I did, so much as the impact I had on other people's lives. One of my past students sent me a book she'd written. She said she included a lot of content related to her work with me, because it was a total turning point for her whole life and catapulted her forward on her journey. I think that's part of a legacy. It touched me, because it made me realise I have made a difference. Sometimes you forget how all of the little things you do can bring about significant changes for the better in people's lives.

### How big a problem is bingeing in our society?

Bingeing is a huge problem. Alcohol, in particular, is seen as a social glue. Instead of initiating young boys into manhood using a meaningful and empowering ritual, they're given a drink of alcohol on their birthday as some kind of sign they're now an adult. What kind of initiation is encouraging your kid to drink? And it often includes the girls as well. Research now shows that the younger a person is when they have their first drink, the more likely they are to become addicted, and the more difficult it is to give it up.

One of my clients said his dad gave him his first drink when he was seven, and he drank a whole bottle. A man from one of my *Beat the Binge* classes said his brother died of an overdose of ice, and that his own son, who was only in his late teens, had a problem with alcohol. Still, the man insisted he himself didn't have a problem, even though he admitted to doing methamphetamine once every two weeks, taking a week to recover and smoking dope regularly.

I said, "Well, what about alcohol? Do you drink? He said, "Oh yeah, of course I drink." You know, as if that's a given. I asked him how often he drank, and he said he didn't drink very much. Just three or four times a week...but he doesn't have a drug problem.

A question I'm often asked is what the difference is between someone who just goes out to have a good time and someone who's an alcoholic. My answer is, "One drink. You just don't know which drink it's going to be."

There are people who drink every weekend and think that if they can take some time off, they're not addicted. I once had this client, a high-flying executive who could go three months without a drink, so she said she didn't have a problem. However, she also admitted that most of the time she wouldn't answer the phone at night, because she would slur her words. To put it another way, she was a functional addict. There are a lot of functional addicts in society.

**How do you define bingeing, and when does it become a problem? Is it the repeated behaviour?**

For me, bingeing is taking an excess of something in one sitting, to the point the body can't handle it. If you do that repeatedly, the body comes to regard the excesses as normal. In other words, you're training it to be able to take on more and more.

With most drugs, including alcohol, people often don't realise they're addicted and are attempting to numb the pain they feel inside. Often they don't even comprehend they're in pain. Society has conditioned them to believe they can deal with it by taking a pill, and if it's only done occasionally, they don't have a problem. The truth is that having a break does give the body time to recover, but it hasn't healed the underlying urge to do it again, and again ... and again. As the saying goes, *Repetition is the mother of skill.*

I think there are a number of reasons people binge, but I believe the main one is they want to comfort themselves, and they've never learnt to self-soothe or how to deal with their inner struggles effectively without self-medicating.

**Do you mean an event happened in their life they can't get over or that they're just not happy in life, and this is the way they cover it up?**

It could be a one-off event or something that happened so regularly it became "normal". I think people use all sorts of means to cover up their unhappiness. For example, one of my first clients, who's given me permission to tell her story, was a kleptomaniac. She didn't touch a drop of drink or any other drug. Stealing was her drug. She said she would go into a store, get her adrenals going and steal something. Then she'd come out, throw whatever she'd stolen into the bin and away she'd go to the next store. She didn't even want the object she stole. She was just after the hit. When we dug deeper, I found out she was sexually abused from the age of two.

Something happens to a person, and they frame it in terms of a belief about themselves, which is that they're bad, ugly, stupid and unwanted, and nobody could ever possibly love them. They believe they can never do anything right. What they need to do is reframe the incident in a way that allows them to move forward. I did it by changing the fundamental structures in my life and became a much better version of me, regardless of all the "bad" things I'd done. This is called transcendence, and it's possible for everyone.

### How does your business help these people? What kind of programs do you have?

We assist people in raising their awareness about what they've done, without condoning the behaviour or making them feel wrong about it. After all, if they'd known better, chances are they would have done something better.

As far as my programs go, I have a do-it-yourself (DIY) program, which means you get all of the tools you'll need to raise your awareness and reach the stage where you can significantly cut back on or eliminate whatever you're bingeing on or addicted to.

Now, for people who need a little bit more help, they can do the online *Beat the Binge* program, which is live, so they can ask questions, and it's reinforced by a video program. There are also more intensive three and six-month programs.

There's a five week face-to-face program mainly for people who live in Adelaide or who want to fly in. I also train people to be coaches, so

I'm looking for those who want to help transform lives, their own and others, and do it in a deep and meaningful way. I guess my training isn't for the faint-hearted.

### How does your training help people?

I have created a modality called *Wholistic Psychonomy*. It's a combination of various approaches to healing including breathwork, coaching, counselling and assisting the client to restructure their lives in such a way that the focus is on recognising the body's own healing and recovery potential regarding what works rather than what doesn't anymore. After all, the past is over. What can we do to assist someone in moving forward into a new way of thinking, feeling and being? That's what Wholistic Psychonomy focuses on.

The modality is designed for people to do for both personal and professional development. I cover every major area in life. If a person wants to become a practitioner, I include a huge toolbox of skills to assist them.

We cover empowerment, belief systems, what drives someone and what they can do to transform those belief systems; how to live by design rather than by default. We cover the role the in-utero experience and actual birth play in determining some of the patterns that are employed later in life. For instance, drugs are used in the birthing process, so isn't it obvious that if drugs are associated with survival, you're then going to seek a drug to feel okay later on? That's not rocket science. It's just common sense.

One of the modules is called *Communicating for Success*. I'm keen to teach people the science and art of communicating with others, including those going through difficulties, and being able to assist them in gaining insight. We explore the rules of communication that allow us to delve deeply and quickly, so the client can re-evaluate their lives and make their own decisions. Nothing is imposed from without.

Even though they say you can change a habit in twenty-one days, my experience tells me that deeply ingrained habits, especially addictions where identity issues are involved, need at least three months and one week to make longer-lasting changes. And if they want to have True Choice, then it's one year and one month. This means not forcing the changes but making conscious daily choices and feeling more and more empowered by those choices.

**Does True Choice mean people feel like they have their life back?**

Yes. They know who they are inside. They're no longer this person they become when they've had "a few too many". They're choosing to be who they are, not what their preferred addiction turns them into. People go through a stage where they have their first drink, and they're a bit happy. They become more sociable, because this is their social lubricant. It gives them confidence. Even with other drugs, there's the peer pressure to have the same experience together. If you're not strong in yourself, it's difficult to resist the social acceptance being offered via the drug.

I believe this is the ritual they've set in place, because society offers nothing better. The drugs are made into the monster, which they're not, because a drug is just a drug. Alcohol is just alcohol. It's about what happens when it hits your system. Maybe a person becomes a really violent drunk when they've had too many. They like to go through that nice, happy stage. Then they get to this next phase, where they can either go to sleep or become violent. Different people deal with poison in their body in different ways.

**What about raising awareness?**

In terms of awareness, it's first about the addict admitting they have a problem, because mostly from their point of view, they don't have one. Everybody else has a problem with them. It's a self-centred, selfish point of view and experience, but they're unaware. I think that once their awareness is raised, they can go through the steps where they finally accept they do have a problem, and then they can start the corrective process.

Again, it's not about making them wrong for having taken so long to get to that point. It's more like saying they were a baby, just learning about themselves for the first time, because they hadn't grown up on an emotional level. Then they can continue through the other stages.

**Is there anyone who's come to you that you haven't been able to help?**

The sister of one of my clients came for a session and afterward told my client she didn't believe anything I said. The client said that based on what her sister told her, I'd hit the nail on the head with every one of her sister's issues. My approach evidently didn't work for this woman, and it's as simple as that. I'll admit it. Those who do end up continuing to see me truly are a good match for my methods and ready for transformation. I always do my best to make sure they understand everything is healable.

I'm not everyone's cup of tea, nor are they mine. I often tell my students there are so many in pain waiting for them to learn whatever it is they need to, so they can help these people.

**Do people live in pain?**

Yes. I'm sixty-six years old and working towards dying well, one of my major goals in life. I don't mean dying of old age. I'm planning to die totally healthy. People ask me how I know, and I joke that it's because I'm never going to see a doctor, but in truth I do want it to be a conscious transition, where I'm aware of what's happening.

Right now, I'm watching a few people die and learning from them. I think it's critical to always have an open mind. Being able to facilitate someone to move gracefully through that dying process or major illness is a real privilege. Pain is part of life. Learning to live with it with equanimity is the key. I realise this is easy to say but not necessarily easy to do.

Dying well is more about not being afraid. I've had so much death in my life and so many personal near-death experiences, that I just say, "Meh, it'll be fine." We die in this body, and we live again. Best to keep the body vitally alive while we have it. And for me that means giving it what keeps it healthy: good food, lots of water, exercise... and laughter.

### Regarding your education, can you talk about what you've studied that led you to coaching?

I think I was a teacher from way back. The first class I ever taught was when I was about ten years old. I kept on being put in charge, because I was at a boarding school where a lot of different ages were together, and there weren't enough teachers.

In terms of more formal education, I did an Honours Degree in Psychology. I could have done a master's and a PhD but chose not to, because I thought what was offered at the time was deadly dull. I did a Diploma in Education and went on to also get a Bachelor of Education in Drama, which I think helps in what I've chosen to do.

I trained as a rebirther initially and then did training with Stanislav Grof, who does holotropic breathwork, something I discovered by chance through one of my clients. Holotropic breathwork combines accelerated breathing with provocative music and assists people in entering a non-ordinary state of consciousness. This state activates the natural inner healing process of the individual's psyche. Grof reinforced what I already knew and gave me good structures around the use of music in a breath session.

I'm also a master practitioner of NLP (Neuro-Linguistic Programming). It's the fundamental dynamics between the mind (neuro) and language (linguistic) and how their interplay affects your body and behaviour (programming). I always do some kind of professional development every year, including mainstream and other smaller healing courses, such as pre-Rolfing, which helps me during breath sessions. Rolfing is a system for bringing the human body back into proper alignment.

I've also done Benjamin Harvey's training, because what he's doing is what I unsuccessfully attempted to set up in Adelaide.

Then, of course, there's the University of Life, which gives you all of these experiences, because I've never had a client tell me something I was shocked by. Basically, I'm told I'm un-shockable.

**Do you feel like you're doing what you were meant to do?**

Yes. I knew it when I went for my first breath session at the age of thirty-four. My second husband asked me how I'd become so successful, and I said it's because I just do whatever it takes. I think every little bit you do makes a difference in somebody else's life.

**How can other people find their passion?**

As I keep saying to my younger son, just follow your heart.

Patterns are so strong. Do you want to follow someone else, or could you do something that reflects your gifts? So, follow your heart and have courage, because I know, in every cell of my being, that the work I take people through is courageous work. We're going to be launching Courageous Conversations, which is a little radio/podcast spot where people can share their story, because all of us have these amazing stories to tell.

I think telling your story is one of the key components of healing. It gets a bit lost in the world of entertainment. People think their story isn't as big or interesting, so why bother telling it? In actual fact, every person has a story that deserves to be heard.

**Once you've helped people reach a point where they feel satisfied with bingeing issues, do you continue working with them?**

Absolutely. This is when the real fun starts. I think what happens is that because people are hurt in some way or suffer from a trauma when they're younger, they make it mean something. Once we help them unpack it and see what they really want to do, we can assist them to move forward towards that instead of always dwelling in the past.

*Is your passion the same as your purpose?*

No. You can be passionate about so many things, but is it your purpose? Probably not. I believe purpose is something that evolves. I don't talk much about a life purpose, because I believe it's revealed as you go along, and that if you ever think you have only one purpose and don't continue to have an open mind, you can get locked into something that may or may not be it. I'm not saying you shouldn't be purposeful or have a plan, but if you keep focusing on that one purpose, you may be unaware of all of the other signs that could be leading towards something you would never have even dreamed of.

*Why is mindset important?*

When you understand you're not your mind, then you know you need to be in command of it, rather than it being in command of you. Everyone thinks they're thinking. Mostly you have thoughts that go around and around. How can they be corralled into some kind of order, so you can get to get to a higher level? Einstein said, and I'm paraphrasing here, that you can't solve a problem on the same level as you created it.

To get to the next level, you need to work on mindset. If you're constantly thinking of ways to make your pain disappear, either consciously or unconsciously, by using an activity or drug, then your mind is always going to be clouded, and the real problem is that you don't know it's clouded. As they say, *Energy flows where your focus goes.*

### How do you work on mindset?

I do daily meditation in order to go beyond the mind. I've been meditating for over thirty years. I can do it by sitting in a meditative position or as I go about my life. Hanging out the clothes or digging in the garden can be just as meditative as sitting in lotus. I still believe that part of the meditative process is consciously clearing the mind, because that's the basic necessity in terms of the beginnings of meditation. Having said that, it's not about not having a thought, because that doesn't ever happen. Well, rarely. You might have moments where you believe you have no thoughts, but if you're thinking about it, you're having a thought. Do you see what I mean?

### Do you have any other daily rituals that keep you in peak form?

I eat mostly organic. I have a garden, so I can pick my own vegetables and herbs. I make sure I do at least some form of exercise daily and stand when I work. I rarely sit during the day. I also do mindful breathing exercises every day, and some of those exercises are in a book I wrote, called *Wake Up and Breathe.*

### What other books have you written, and why did you write them?

I wrote my first book. *Your Drug or Your Life*, because my older son at the time was having a major problem with substance abuse.

Just look at the news. I really believe we're taking a punitive approach, which evidently doesn't work. If a child does something naughty, you take them aside and have a chat about what they did wrong, ask them what they could do differently for a better outcome for everyone and set clear boundaries. Instead we say, "You step over this line, and you're going to get punished." As I tell people who hit their kids, violence begets violence. Personally, I've never found physical violence to have an empowering, lasting effect.

In the 1920s there were drugs that were available over the counter, including opiates and amphetamines. People only took them when they needed them. They rarely, if ever, became addicted. There's a book written by Johann Hari called *Chasing the Scream*, and it's the most brilliant exposition on the war on drugs I've seen.

*Your drug or your life* means having to choose between them, because the drug will take your life. There's a saying in AA that I think is accurate. The person takes a drink, and then after a little while the drink takes the drink, and then after a little while the drink takes the person. I don't have anything against alcohol or any other drug. Like I say to my sons, I don't have to wake up in your body. I don't have to deal with the thoughts you're having or feel how you feel the morning after. And there's always a morning after...unless there isn't.

I also co-authored a book with a friend of mine. It's called *Angels in Hell*. The idea came up as we were travelling to the Gold Coast by train. It turns out we'd both been sexually assaulted when we were younger. We had so many similarities that I suggested we write a book, so we did. It was mainly to help people understand that whatever happens to them it doesn't affect who they are inside. During my experience I realised that no one could hurt who I was on the inside. That's what I walked away with, before I'd ever done any inner work. I just knew I had an inner strength no one could violate.

***You come across as someone who is accepting and nonjudgmental, regardless of a person's situation. How do you do that?***

Part of the whole process of healing is to understand that people do what they do, because that's the best they can do. They don't have any other way of behaving, otherwise they would. I think some people believe in pure evil. Well, I've met a lot of bad people in my time, but I wouldn't label them that way. They've just done bad things. I seem to have this ability to look past whatever their behaviour is and into their souls to see who they really are. I think that's part of what I offer in my trainings and classes, because that's all I'm doing the whole time. Or at least doing my best to do....a gift from my parents.

I think we need lots of people who are willing to be courageous and face up to whatever difficulties they're having. Then they need to be able to move through them and help others do the same.

 To discover more about how Ruby can help you *Elevate Your Health*, visit

www.elevate-books.com/health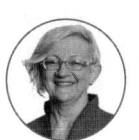

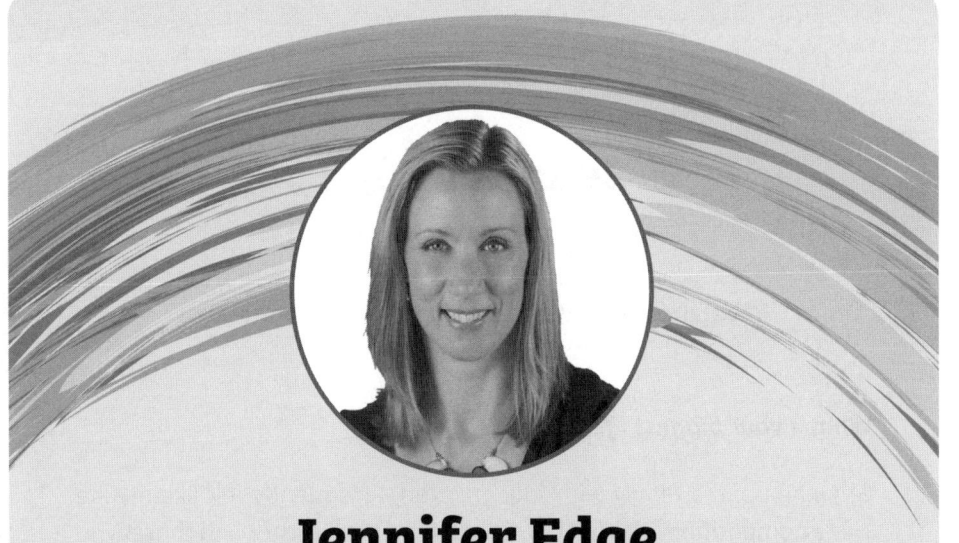

# Jennifer Edge

## Master Your Mindset

Jennifer Edge is a certified life coach, presenter and has over ten years of experience as a physiotherapist. She's particularly interested in the connection between mindset and its impact on quality of life.

Having been a competitive rower for over twelve years, Jennifer understands the importance of mindset training. Her unique style of coaching and training utilises the effective yet simple strategies that athletes routinely use to reach peak physical and mental balance. Her belief is that you don't have to be a professional athlete to learn these tools and apply them in any area of life for permanent, positive changes.

Jennifer specializes in helping professionals, athletes, parents and students achieve their true potential by prioritizing their health and wellbeing. She's the founder of Symetrica and is passionate about working with people to help them rebalance the connection between mind, body and spirit, thus enabling them to be their true self and live the most spectacular life.

# Jennifer Edge

## Master Your Mindset

### Rebalance your Mind, Body and Spirit Connection

**What's your biggest life lesson?**

Growing up in a family with four children, I frequently felt like my life was a competition. Against my older brothers, my sister and those who participated with me or against me in all of the sports I played. I loved sport, and I was a good athlete. This quickly became my way of getting attention and love from my parents, particularly my father. Winning was my ticket to feeling important and special. It became my measuring stick for feeling loved and accepted. Over time, my need for external approval and acceptance led to relying on external achievement and others to make me happy.

Five years ago, I suffered a major identity crisis. My mindset and body were completely out of balance, and as a result my performance in every area of my life started to suffer. I was in a job I hated, flailing in a dysfunctional relationship I'd stayed in for years longer than I deserved and was binge eating until I felt sick, I had distanced myself from family and friends, and all of this left me feeling completely worthless.

I eventually ended that five-year relationship, quit my job and moved back to Australia after living in England for almost five years. This led me on a journey of self-discovery. I felt this gut-wrenching void inside of me. I gradually began to realise that all my life I'd constantly felt like I had to prove my worth, not just to others but also to myself. Because of my lack of self-awareness, I continued to try and fill it, unsuccessfully, through external means. I would immerse myself in work, become needy for love and approval in relationships, buy clothes and shoes, escape on a holiday, seek achievement in sport, eat comfort food and distract myself with television. Anything to try and fill the huge void. Not only was this causing me severe depression, but it also resulted in accumulating large credit card debt, deteriorating health and wellbeing and a non-existent social life.

In 2012, a friend introduced me to personal development, and it's been a life-changing experience. Along this journey, I discovered life and wellness coaching, which gave me a light at the end of a long, dark tunnel. What I learnt about myself, and the coaching skills I acquired, have helped me transform my life. I've developed a level of self-awareness, self-belief and self-worth that has allowed me to steer a new course towards creating what I truly want and deserve in my life.

I started to develop self-awareness and came to realise that I was the only one who could fill the void inside of me. Because I had ignored the signs from my heart/intuition, my mind, body, and even the universe, were giving me feedback that I was off course in my life. I started to listen to the feedback and applied the coaching strategies I'd learnt. This resulted in deepening my self-belief and self-worth and a desire to transform my life. I discovered that the secret to having a fulfilling life starts from the inside, which can then be projected into the external world.

### What's the one message you wish to share with the world?

I truly believe that the life you have is a reflection of what you believe you deserve. You have the power to create the life you want, no ifs, buts or maybes. There's proof out there it's possible. Other people are doing it, and doing it with integrity. What's holding you back are the limits you put on yourself. You sell yourself short and stay inside of your comfort bubble. I want you to know you're worthy of an amazing life. I believe the way to achieve it is to start with self awareness and then expand that awareness it to your external world. This will allow you to see the obstacles you put in your own way, and once you can identify them, you can overcome them.

How badly do you want it? Are you willing to burst your comfort bubble? Are you willing to let go of the beliefs that are holding you back from the life you deserve? Are you open to a new way of thinking and feeling? Stop looking for answers out in the world. They're inside you.

### *What decisions have made a difference in your life?*

1.  Deciding to believe in myself

    I'm the only one who can create the life I want and transform my mind and body to lead a life filled with happiness and fulfilment.

2. Taking responsibility for my life

    No longer blaming other people and experiences for how my life turned out. I've directed the focus inwards, so I could take responsibility for myself and my life. I now try to accept and appreciate that everyone who's played a part in my life did the best they knew how.

3.  Appreciating that I'm not perfect

    Guess what...I'm not perfect! Just like most people, I'm my own worst critic. I learnt to appreciate that I'm an imperfect person and let go of the expectation of being perfect. The illusion of perfection cripples progression. It took me a long time to accept that it's okay to make mistakes. It's the only way to learn and grow into a better person.

    The most successful people in business and sport are also the ones who've failed the most but are able to learn a lesson from their failures. The difference is that they didn't give up. They used the setbacks as learning tools to improve and trained themselves to be resilient and overcome failures.

> "I've missed more than 9000 shots in my career. I've lost almost 300 games. 26 times, I've been trusted to take the game winning shot and missed. I've failed over and over and over again in my life. And that is why I succeed.
> ~ *Michael Jordan*

4.  Becoming vulnerable

    Being vulnerable is essential to creating the life I want. I believe that vulnerability is a sign of inner strength. When you're being vulnerable, you're valuing who you are as a person. Vulnerability ensures I'm able to create the best relationships, career, and wellbeing, and be the most authentic version of myself.

5.  Giving myself permission to change

    To create momentum, all I needed was a series of small actions that resulted in permanent, positive change. Taking risks is scary, but on the other end of the risk are the most amazing rewards. I didn't let the little voice in my head stop me from doing what I wanted and needed to be happy.

    To truly believe in myself, I couldn't give up on creating and living the life I desired. I closed the gap between thinking and doing, because success is only achieved when you move through discomfort and take action. The more discomfort, the greater the victory.

5.  Letting go of judgment and expectation of myself and others

    I consciously work on replacing expectation with intention. I decide on my intention each day, rather than having a preconceived idea as to what should happen or be said/felt in different situations. This allows me to no longer get caught up in the anxiety and tension I used to feel. As a result, any frustration and disappointment I may feel is drastically reduced or gone completely. I feel so much more balanced in my emotions, which has helped me be kinder not only to others but to myself.

6.    Treating each person as a whole

Having been a physiotherapist for over ten years, I've focused on treating people with physical pain and injuries. I realized I wanted to do more, so now I help people transform other areas of their life as well. I've seen firsthand how developing a person's mindset can drastically alter the course of their life and set them on a path towards fulfilment and happiness.

**What's your biggest WHY?**

I consistently had that niggling feeling at the end of the day, when my mind was quiet, that something wasn't right...something was missing. This motivated me to explore more about the connection between the mind, body and spirit and how an imbalance or asymmetry can result in disastrous consequences.

What I love most about my work is that I get to connect with a variety of people every day. It gives me a greater sense of purpose. I want more people to develop unwavering self-belief and self worth. When this happens, they will realise they're powerful beyond measure. There's no stopping them from taking the actions they need to create a deeply fulfilling life.

Consider this: people are living longer, are richer and have more choices than ever before. But as a society we're the most in debt, overweight, medicated and addicted than ever before.

Why are people doing this to themselves?

It usually comes down to daily lifestyle choices. Most people live in a state of unconsciousness and aren't self-aware enough to even know they're unhappy or that they're neglecting their health and wellbeing. One of the most important lessons I learnt from Brené Brown is that people numb themselves.

But the bad news is you can't selectively numb feelings, so you end up numbing both the good and bad ones. As a consequence, you try to find solace through external means. But that little unfulfilled feeling keeps coming up, so you continue to try and block it out by working harder, buying more things, eating more food, drinking more or zoning out with TV or the internet.

The cycle continues, unless you're able to wake up! You alone have the power to move out of this mindset and release yourself from your current state. I like to look at it as if everyone has two choices:

1.  To continue on the path they're on (and suffer the consequences)

OR

2.  To develop their awareness and learn effective strategies (and change what isn't working).

It's your life, it's your choice.

To put it simply, I want to inspire people. I want them to look me in the eye and say, "Because of you, I didn't settle. Because of you, I didn't quit."

**What are you passionate about?**

I'm passionate about working with people to reach new heights in their life through transformation of their mind, body and spirit. I've often witnessed people who have blinkers on. They work themselves into the ground whilst neglecting the other areas of their life. As a result, instead of being rewarded for all of their hard work and being able to enjoy life doing what they love, such as travelling the world to experience different cultures, spending precious time with loved ones, having fun with friends or even creating a charity, their time and money are spent addressing the health and relationship issues they now suffer from.

To put it in a scientific way, the human body is designed to maintain a state of homeostasis, meaning internal equilibrium. This is where all of the systems of the body work together in a balancing act. The mind and body are constantly giving you feedback to let you know when you're out of balance. Unfortunately, if you lack self-awareness or don't value yourself, you won't recognise the signs of being out of balance. Then you may not be willing to do what you must to make the necessary changes to bring yourself back into balance and start living more true to you.

When you're in a state of imbalance for an extended period of time, your body will continue to try and compensate by giving you signs. What's interesting is that if you choose to ignore the signs, they become more and more obvious. For example, it may start like being hit with a feather. Then if you don't change your actions, your body will up the ante and hit you with a brick. If you still choose to ignore the signs, a truck will come hurtling towards you. Then you're in real trouble.

Here's an example I've seen time and time again. A person is hugely successful in their business and putting in a load of extra time to progress it even further. They're earning an absolute packet, and the business is growing so fast it's hard to keep up. They need to employ more staff to meet with the demand. Their hard work is paying off, and they're able to buy a big house in a nice suburb and send their two children to the top private schools.

Everything seems to be going so well... but if you scratch beneath the surface you'll see the truth.

- Their health is suffering, because they're stressed all of the time.

- They sleep so poorly, they're pretty much an insomniac.

- They don't make time to exercise or eat healthy meals and generally eat on the run. This means highly processed, high sugar, high fat and low quality food.

- When they do spend time with their family, they're unable to connect. This is because they're either distracted by the huge workload hanging over their head or are so exhausted they don't have the energy to engage.

The end result is their health starts to deteriorate, they end up in hospital after a heart attack, they have Type 2 diabetes due to being overweight and they're on a variety of medication to treat their ailments and illnesses. To top it off, their partner decides they're not happy, because they feel neglected and want a divorce. *"But things were going so well"*, they think. *"I don't understand what went wrong."* This is a classic case of a lack of awareness leading to a complete imbalance in their life.

My mission is to help people from all walks of life create more self-worth through self-awareness and to ultimately assist them in expanding that awareness into their external world. They can then make the changes they need to ensure they're in an ultimate state of wellbeing. As a coach I guide people through the steps they need to take to bring about true long-lasting transformation, so they can uncover their inner strength.

"Whether you think you can or you think you can't, you're right".
*~ Henry Ford*

When you take back control of your health, your career, your relationship, your time and your finances, you ultimately take back control of your life. I know as well as anyone that you can't control everything in your life, and you can't control other people. But you can control your responses, thoughts, feelings, decisions and actions. Life and wellness coaching provides you with the support and skills to accomplish this. You're able to utilize these skills every day and draw upon them in challenging situations. Through coaching, I facilitate my clients to find their own answers and provide an environment in which they feel safe to be vulnerable, honest and their true self. A relationship is formed where they're heard and understood.

I want to see you getting out there and taking a chance on yourself. No one else is going to back you, unless you do it first. It's scary that the vast majority of people play it safe, but what's really sad about the situation is you can still fail at something that's not fulfilling to you. So why not take a chance on yourself and live life the way you truly want? Believe in yourself enough to get outside your comfort bubble. In fact...burst your comfort bubble!

**What do you think people's biggest issues are?**

▶ **They don't know or believe in themselves**

I've experienced a lot of people who say they don't like personal development and coaching. Why wouldn't you want to transform into your best self? Yes, it's all about you, because you're the only one who will be there your whole life. You were there at the beginning and you'll be there all the way to the end. If you can create a better version of yourself starting with self-awareness, then you will be a better partner, colleague, friend, parent, sibling, and child. Just a better person overall. Your external world is just a reflection of your internal world, so if you're not happy with yourself or don't love and believe in yourself, then your life will mirror this thought process.

Elevate Your Health

► **Fear**

Fear prevents people from living the life they deserve. Some say it's a fear of failure, but I believe it's a fear of success that prevents them from taking action. For instance, fear of the unknown. "Who will I be when I'm successful?" "Will people treat me differently?" "Where will I fit in then?" Fear is a part of life. Fear is built into your DNA to protect you, but it can also run your life if you let it. What a lot of people don't realise is that courage is not the absence of fear. People who are courageous still feel the fear, but they take risks and live outside of their comfort zone, because they believe they deserve a better life.

> "Do the one thing you think you cannot do. Fail at it. Try again. Do better the second time. The only people who never tumble are those who never mount the high wire. This is your moment. Own it."
>
> ~ *Oprah Winfrey*

► **Lack of vulnerability**

Vulnerability is a sign of strength, not weakness. It's putting yourself out there, even when you're afraid of what could happen. Being vulnerable can result in achieving even more success in your career, having a stronger and deeper connection with your spouse and being a better parent. It also means having a deeper sense of self-worth, a superior level of health and wellness and creating more wealth. All of this will help you have the freedom to live the life of your dreams.

▶ **Holding on to the past**

Most people walk around holding onto so much from their past, it's like dragging around a heavy weight behind them. It tends to be a mixture of guilt, shame, fear and judgement. This can prevent you moving forward in life. If you could learn from the past and then let go of it, you could stop sabotaging yourself and progress faster.

> "When you get to a place where you understand that love and belonging, your worthiness, is a birthright and not something you have to earn, anything is possible."
> ~ Brene Brown

***Do you have an approach to your mindset and wellness coaching?***

I draw upon my strong background in competitive sport and my extensive experience and knowledge of the connection of mind and body to help my clients achieve the best results. The most successful athletes in the world understand the power of training their mind and body to perform at their peak. You'll also notice that the truly great athletes are the ones who are the most passionate. You don't have to be a world-class athlete to benefit from the same type of simple and effective strategies they use to perform at their best. The good news is they can easily be applied to business, relationships, finances, parenting and other areas, with outstanding outcomes.

For the best results, my clients follow **The Six-Step Desire System**

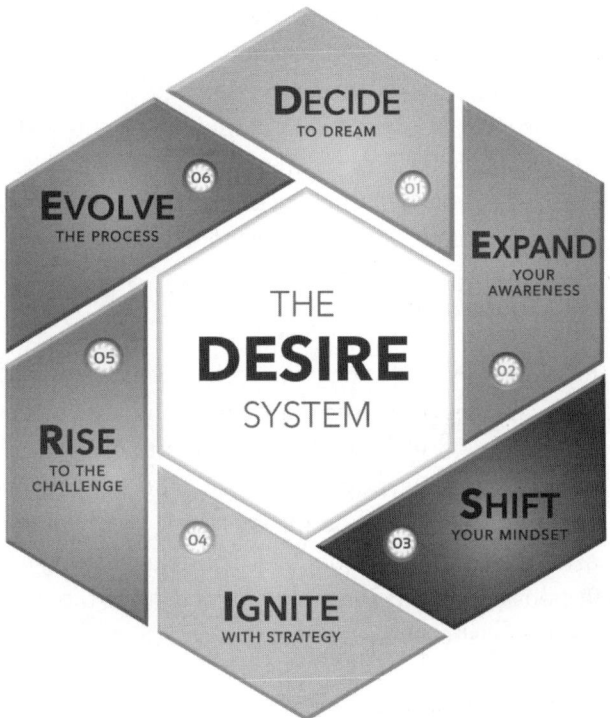

### Step 1:   Decide to Dream

This is when you give yourself permission to dream about how you desire your life to be. You want to allow yourself time to dream bigger than ever before. Ask yourself the question, "What would I do with my life if I couldn't fail?" This is when you take the time to develop your desire to create the life you truly deserve. The kind of life you're worthy of.

### Step 2:  Expand Your Awareness

Developing a greater awareness of self means looking inside your mindset and discovering why and how you think, feel and act and what influences the decisions you make. As Lao Tzu once said, "He who knows others is wise; he who knows himself is enlightened." Identify any problems you may not have been totally aware of and take time to identify any gaps in your skill set. Once you have self-awareness, you can develop awareness of your external world as well.

### Step 3:  Shift Your Mindset

Start to shift your way of thinking and feeling. This is done by making the necessary changes to the problems you identified in step two. It's time to shift your mindset from closed or fixed to one that is open to growing and changing. Dr Wayne Dyer said, "Be open to everything and attached to nothing." You do this by letting go of limiting beliefs, moving past the conditioning from your upbringing, stopping the self-sabotaging behaviours and releasing yourself from the shame, guilt and judgment of past events.

### Step 4:  Ignite With Strategy

This is when you commit to change by creating an effective plan to follow. What is your current system? Is it getting you the results you want in your life? If not, the best way to get the right results is to redesign the system you use.

### Step 5:  Rise to the Challenge

Start putting the plan into action. Those with profound self-worth rise to the challenge, make tough decisions and take risks, because they know they're worthy of the life that lies on the other side of any discomfort they go through. No more playing it small or safe!

**Step 6: Evolve the Process**

This is when you take the actions you've started to perform and make them part of your everyday routine. As Tony Robbins said, "For changes to be of any true value, they've got to be lasting and consistent." Make the necessary changes as you work back through the system. Do you need to dream bigger? Has your dream changed, even slightly? Was there anything you missed?

If you follow this Six-Step Desire System, I guarantee you'll learn the strategies to develop awareness and create profound levels of self-worth that will ensure you make the best decisions, which will result in a life of fulfilment, happiness and success.

I have a multifaceted approach to my life and wellness coaching. I like to serve people in different ways, so I don't limit myself to only one-on-one coaching. Workshops are an integral part of my business, because they provide an environment where groups of likeminded people can come together and learn. It also provides an amazing opportunity for collaborative learning and networking between the participants.

I also have a regular blog that I hope inspires people, because ultimately I'm here to serve others. I want to help people be more active in their approach towards having a greater sense of self-worth that's reflected in their everyday decisions and to assist them in living a life of supreme wellness, fulfilment, happiness and success.

***What courses have you completed that enabled you to get started or build your business?***

I love learning and expanding my knowledge. I've completed a Life Coaching Certification with Authentic Education in Sydney after developing a great interest in human behaviour and psychology, and how mindset influences our lives.

I've also completed a Bachelor of Arts in Human Movement Studies at the University of Technology, Sydney and a Master's Degree in Physiotherapy at The University of Sydney. As a result, I have extensive knowledge and understanding of the human body and mind. I'm completely blown away by the complexity of the human body and how all of the systems work together to allow people to live, learn and grow every day. To improve my knowledge and skills in running a successful business, I've also studied a number of business courses with Authentic Education, including marketing, time management, and sales.

### Why is mindset important?

Training your mindset is hands down the most powerful way to transform yourself, and ultimately your life. You have to be able to leverage your strengths and know your weaknesses in order to give yourself the best shot at living the life you dream of. A lot of people are stuck in the same patterns of behaviour, and they believe it's fixed forever. But I know for a fact this is untrue. If you start by developing self-awareness, you can transform to a growth mindset where nothing is fixed, and you realise you have the power to change the course of your life.

There's an epidemic of people thinking that the way to be happy and *fill the void* is by changing their external environment. This could include having more things, being in a relationship (even a bad one), drinking more, eating too much or staying at a job they hate because the pay is good. I'm proof this doesn't work. It can be a hard pill to swallow, because for a lot of people it's a deeply ingrained habitual pattern they may have been involved in for most of their life.

However, Deepak Chopra's researchers found that forty percent of a person's happiness is based on voluntary choices, fifty percent is genetically determined and ten percent is due to living conditions. If only ten percent of your happiness is dependent on living conditions, it doesn't make sense to keep looking outside of yourself for the answers. You have the power inside of you to make yourself happy and create the life you want.

Your mindset forms the foundation of how you think, feel and act, as well as how you treat yourself and others. To develop a mindset for fulfilment and happiness, you have to be able to navigate the mind.

The three keys to navigating the mind:

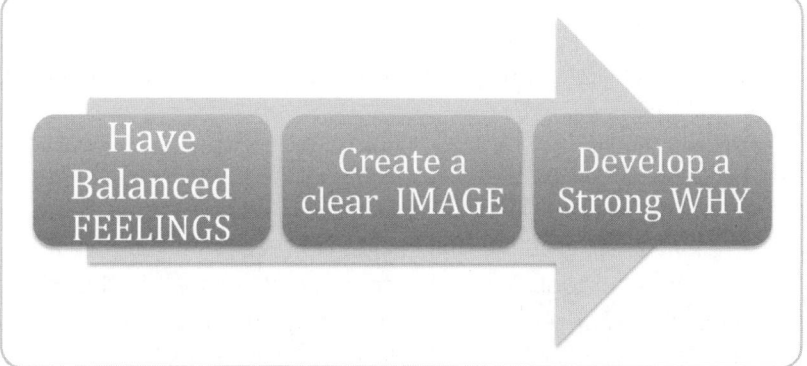

1.   Have *awareness of your feelings* and the ability to *balance* them.

2.   Create a profound *crisp, internal image* of what you want. An image that engages all of the senses.

3.   Develop *a strong reason WHY* for a clear link to your values.

**What are some tools or strategies you could recommend for keeping balance in your life?**

▸   **Meditation**

The benefits of meditation are numerous. They include but are not limited to:

- improved focus

- more clarity

- decreased stress

- being more relaxed

- the ability to be more present

- being more emotionally balanced

- the ability to respond rather than react emotionally to situations

▶ **Imagery**

Creating crisp, vivid internal images of what you want in your life is a powerful tool. Being able to immerse yourself in the scene with all of your senses helps you to stay on course towards your dreams and convinces your body this image is actually your future.

▶ **Live within your values**

Determine what's important to you. What do you truly value in life? Too often people compromise their own needs to please others, leaving them feeling cheated and not good enough. Do you have a values conflict? A mismatch of values may cause internal conflict, anxiety and stress that can prevent you from taking the necessary actions to transform your life.

▶ **List writing**

This tool is incredibly powerful in rewiring neural networks in the brain. The more connections you can make when list writing, the stronger the result. It's a powerful tool in helping deepen your self-worth, self-belief and understanding yourself more.

One of the most powerful lists I learnt through Ben Harvey was writing down a hundred things I love about myself. I found it so difficult to write the first time, because it sounded so narcissistic, but then I realised if I don't love myself, I can't love anyone else the way they deserve. Does that sound like something you could do? Go on, give it a go. Once you finish, you'll feel genuinely fantastic about who you are.

▸ **Goal Setting**

Goal setting is a great way to stay motivated towards what you want. But quite often your goals can seem too big, too difficult and too far away. One of the best suggestions I can make about setting goals is to not overwhelm yourself by setting too many at a time. Everyone tends to process situations in a different way, so goal-setting should be accomplished according to your processing mechanism.

Some people are more linear in their thinking, and therefore one major goal is best to focus on at any one time. Others can think in a more cyclical manner and are able to handle up to three major goals at a time. Another great tip I learnt is that you'll be faced with much less resistance if you can break the goals down into smaller, more achievable steps.

> "If you don't plan your life, other people will plan it for you and what they've got planned for you is not much".
> ~ Jim Rohn

**Do you have a coach or mentor who motivates you?**

Having a coach is essential for keeping me accountable and helping me stay on track with my progress. The sessions help me feel supported, especially when I'm taking on a new challenge in my personal life or business.

When I first started coaching I had a mentor, Rob Mason, I would contact whenever I was faced with new challenges and felt like I needed advice from someone who'd been through it all before. He provided a wealth of knowledge and experience. I also found it reassuring, because he was proof that what I was doing had been done before, so I knew I could achieve what I set my mind to.

Other mentors I draw inspiration from include Tony Robbins, Wayne Dyer, Jim Rohn, Jack Canfield and Jim Carrey. And of course I want to thank Benjamin J Harvey and Authentic Education for being such an amazing teacher and support throughout my learning process. I'm consistently inspired by the journey my mentors have been on and the message they convey to help change the world.

### How can people become their own success story?

What I tell my coaching clients is, you don't need to prove your worth to anyone. You don't need to be perfect or ashamed of who you are, because you're worthy of happiness, love and acceptance. You deserve to be successful and have a loving relationship. You deserve to have a life of fulfilment, happiness and wellbeing in order to go out and be the most successful version of yourself.

You're just as special and important as anyone else. You're worthy of a great life just because you're you.

 To discover more about how Jennifer can help you *Elevate Your Health*, visit

www.elevate-books.com/health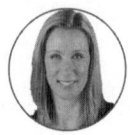

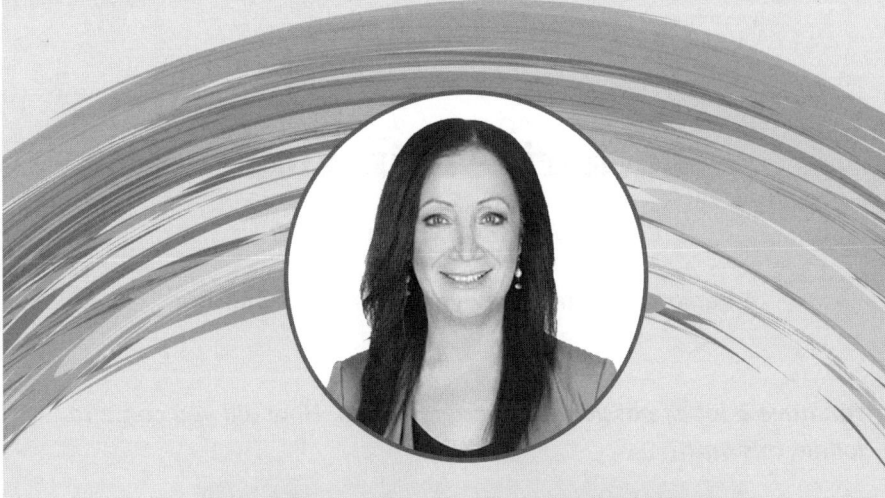

# Catherine Printziou
## Energy Healing Unveiled

Catherine was introduced to and mentored about the healing arts by her grandmother, a Greek refugee, who was a renowned healer, midwife and soothsayer.

Catherine studied Western herbal medicine and joined the National Herbalist Association of Australia in 2000. She studied *Ayurveda* in India, that included treatments and *Ayurvedic* massage. She's a yoga and meditation teacher and uses yoga therapies such as *pranayama* and meditation in her healing programs. She also uses energy healing methods such as crystal wands and energy psychotherapy, taught to her by great masters in Australia, India and Tibet.

Catherine has taken her knowledge and used it to develop comprehensive healing programs based on Ancient Greek principles that take place in intense energy locations.

Besides healing, Catherine's passion is teaching. She loves sharing her knowledge in a simple and caring way in order to guide and empower people to be their own healer.

# Catherine Printziou

## Energy Healing Unveiled

### A Personal Journey of Revelations and Expansion

***You have a lot of passion for energy healing. How did you come to follow this path?***

Well, I love the unseen. The magic and mysteries of life. I grew up with this reality, as my paternal grandmother was a renowned healer. She was of Greek heritage and grew up in Turkey but due to the political situation there was forced to flee to Greece in 1922, only taking what she could carry. However, what she also had were her skills, knowledge and experience in the occult. In Greece she developed a reputation as a healer, midwife and soothsayer. Even when she came to Sydney in 1970, people who knew of her from Greece would come knocking on our door, looking for her. I grew up with healing and the supernatural being as common as watching television after school. She influenced me both actively and passively.

However, I put that aside and followed the Western education system. I studied hard and received a university scholarship and two university degrees and followed an academic path in Linguistics and Education. It seemed an achievement at the time, but several years later I felt dissatisfied. This kind of mental energy didn't feed my soul, and I realized I was off course from my life purpose.

It's fortunate that in 1998 I had the option of taking a redundancy from my government job in curriculum writing, and I jumped at the opportunity to study Western herbal medicine. I was overjoyed to learn remedies from nature and how and why they work, but I also realised we were only treating the symptoms of disease, albeit in a more natural way, and not the disease itself.

 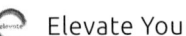

Thanks to my incredible teachers, the generation before me who fought long and hard to legalise herbal medicine in Australia, I was directed to study energy healing. Here was my missing link to getting explanations that quenched my logical and illogical mind. Now I could understand what my grandmother was saying and doing, and this legitimised what I already knew.

Let me say again there needs to be an understanding of certain basic principles before you can comprehend energy healing and how it works. Once you own this knowledge, and it makes sense to you, there's no turning back. Your truth has changed and expanded, so of course you'll want to learn more. In my case, I wanted to learn everything. When you have a revelation, you get an incredible rush, a hunger, and you want to uncover more.

My journey continued to India, where I studied, tried and practised *Ayurvedic* medicine, which is one of the world's oldest holistic healing systems developed there thousands of years ago. It's based on the belief that health and wellness depend on a delicate balance between the mind, body and spirit. *Ayurvedic* medicine focuses on good health, rather than fighting disease.

I also studied Theta Healing, where brainwaves are put into a theta state, and you can even alter the structure of DNA. I learned energy healing using a crystal wand that magnifies the energy utilised for healing by up to six-hundred percent. These crystals have been formed in the depths of the earth from lava and compressed for thousands or millions of years. They're full of energy that can be directed to perform energy healing. Remember, we're one with everything in our universe, made of the same ingredients. Therefore, everyone can unite with and direct this energy to alter its current state, manipulate its particles and restore themselves to health.

So I started off as an herbalist, then an energy healer, and kept adding more modalities to assist my patients. In 2003 I was drawn to discover the culture of my ancestors, so I moved back to Greece where I lived for eight years. The energy was amazing. I felt the nature, light, colours and vibrations as I walked around archaeological sites. I spent endless summers on the islands, swimming in crystal clear waters, eating wholesome, unprocessed food and going to high-energy locations to recharge my batteries.

This was a significant phase of my journey. It was in Greece where I discovered the missing component to my healing, or perhaps all healings: the environment. As I keep saying, we're all connected. Our particles interact with what's around us, and we exchange energies, so it's potent to exchange high-frequency energy from a pristine, natural environment where great minds and healers have left their energetic imprints. In this type of environment I performed the most amazing healings. They were more intense. Changes were rapid, and patients were transformed.

### This is a broad and elusive question, but what is energy healing?

To answer that, I have to first clarify what energy is, because it's been used quite liberally to describe many things. The Cambridge Dictionary defines energy as the power and ability to be physically and mentally active. It's the capacity of a physical system to do work. Eastern esoteric definitions see energy as a life force. In both definitions, energy is a living force that creates movement, actions and life. Without energy, there's no life.

In physics if any living or non-living object is dissected to its smallest unit, it comes down to the atom, which is just particles of orbiting light, composed of electrons that are particles of light with a negative charge, while protons are particles of light with a positive charge, and neutrons are particles of light with no charge. So in fact, all animate and inanimate objects are compacted particles of light.

Another simple fact from physics is that light, when dissected by refracting it through a prism, is made up of four primary colours with blending variations between them. Colours have been scientifically shown to contain different frequencies, or wavelengths, of light and therefore contain different qualities. This is important to understand, because energy healers manipulate each colour in the energy healing process and use the qualities and frequencies of the colour to achieve the desired outcome in energy healing.

For example, the grounding root chakra is primarily red, a low frequency colour that connects everyone to the earth's energies. As you move up the chakra system to the highest chakra at the top of the head, the colour is primarily electric white-violet, the highest, finest frequency. This connects you to the divine, or universal, source.

Another scientific fact is that ninety-eight percent of the world is made up of six main elements: hydrogen, nitrogen, oxygen, carbon, phosphorus and calcium. The other two percent is made up of trace quantities of the remaining eighty-six elements, which makes it ninety two in total. So most of what you see around you is made up of these six main elements. The only difference is the bonds that hold them together. Everything is made up of the same substances, physically and energetically. If this is true, it makes sense that by manipulating these energies, the condition and composition, or frequency, can be altered. This means the health of the person being treated can also be altered.

### What real implications does this have for us?

Knowledge shouldn't be just for the sake of knowing. It needs to be applied. If the planet is made up of the same substances everyone is made from, meaning different frequencies of light, then the notion of unity and oneness should be easy to comprehend. Humans aren't isolated beings but are connected to each other, as well as the environment. In that case, it's important to choose carefully who and what you connect to and exchange energy particles with.

You might notice you experience different energies when in the middle of a dirty, polluted city as opposed to clean and pristine natural environments. Or when surrounded by people who drain your energy as opposed to those who leave you feeling happy and energized. You're constantly exchanging energy with everything around you. There's no boundary line to isolate the physical body from the rest of the world. Everyone gives and takes energy from each other and from the environment in positive and/or negative doses.

Using this understanding, an energy healer can become a channel and remove energy from a person or body part, while also directing clean, healthy energy to replace it. By becoming a channel, the healer doesn't use their own energy and become depleted and eventually sick. They use the universal energy, be it earth's from below or divine from above, as is needed for the patient's condition. This means it's possible to remove or add energy to assist in a patient's healing. I say this from personal experience. It's the quickest way to see any change in a person's condition. Sometimes it can be instantaneous.

Another cornerstone for healers is that energy follows intention. You put a thought or command into this energy, and it must obey. It will carry your command, because it's a Law of the Universe. In this way, negative thoughts or curses, as well as healing, can be transmitted. Energy has been deemed the 4-D Reality. It consists of a frequency or vibration of your own energy that originates from a thought, so pay attention to your thoughts. Be aware of what you're thinking. You can heal with your thought energy, or you can create disease in the same way. Your thoughts penetrate and influence your energy.

In reality, humans aren't only made up of circulatory, digestive, lymphatic, and nervous systems but also the invisible, magical, incredible energy system. It penetrates all body systems and when used effectively can influence and heal all diseased body parts. This energy system consists of the *auric* field, which are the layers of energy that surround you and all things that connect everyone to each other, and chakras, which are energy stations at different parts of the body that distribute energy to surrounding organs. There are major and minor chakras at the front and back of the body (each organ has at least one minor chakra of its own), as well as energy meridians that connect these energy centres and allow the energy to flow throughout the body.

Thus, when energy healers *see* or *feel* a patient's energy, either clairvoyantly or by specialized photography, they notice the different colours that surround the patient and penetrate them. Using this method, healers can analyse the state of a patient's physical body and by the flow of their energy see where stagnation and blocks are occurring. Diseased parts are generally darker and duller in colour and don't have a fine, vibrating flow.

This is a great diagnostic tool, because healers can catch and prevent a disease that's visible on the energy body before it penetrates into the physical body. For example, a person doesn't feel well, so they go to the doctor, have tests done, and everything comes back negative. Then within a short time, usually a matter of months, they have a major disease. They could feel it in their energy body before it had manifested in their physical body.

**You've explained in a clear and simple way how energy healing can repair the physical body, but what role does it have on psychological issues?**

It plays a huge and effective therapeutic role. A psychological shock, trauma, major disappointment or hurt first shows up in a person's aura as a dark energy, or scar, in their *auric* field. If left untreated it grows energetically, especially if it's constantly fed by thoughts of the trauma.

This will gradually penetrate the *auric* layers, enter the chakras, and then the physical body, and manifest as disease in different body parts.

There are many examples of people getting physically ill following major emotional trauma. For example, research has correlated sorrow and heart disease, anger and liver disease, and fears with kidney malfunctions.

Dark, energetic scarring can also disturb a person's emotional/ psychological state. Talking about it is helpful, but it shouldn't stop there. By obsessively thinking and talking about this trauma, it grows and develops an energy of its own and takes over in the form of phobias, depression or suicidal tendencies. This traumatic energy needs to be removed, and the gap it creates needs to be filled with a positive visualisation, or the thought will return.

The trauma can be removed energetically by the healer, or the person experiencing the emotional pain, by a ritual of forgiveness and letting go and replacing it with a positive visualisation of how they'd like the situation to have turned out. This can be easier said than done, because if someone is immersed in their emotional pain, it's difficult to remain objective and rise above it. If it's beyond their capability, they may need help from an energy healer to remove the trauma before it enters the physical body and starts the spiral of disease or disturbs them on an emotional/psychological level.

### What are some personal revelations you've experienced along your journey?

I've had many personal realizations and revelations along the way. The key is to be open and alert to receive them, and when an unusual occurrence happens, to know there's a message to be received. The answer may not come for some time, but be open to receive it when it does.

Most people are oblivious to messages, because they're too busy with their rushed lives. Something extraordinary happens, but they give it a quick thought and a "Wow" before brushing it aside and forgetting about it. There needs to be an openness to expanding knowledge and awareness of the cause and effect of what's happening around you. It's necessary in order to understand the more abstract, yet real, occurrences in your life and to further expand your truths.

There are some general revelations I'd like to share that illustrate the expansion of knowledge and truth. Imagine if a detective investigating a crime finds evidence that leads them to arrest Person A. The detective is sure this person committed the crime. However, other evidence comes to light that Person B did it. By uncovering this new evidence, their truth has now changed. People also tend to operate like this. They have certain truths and beliefs upon which they base their life, but when more evidence comes to light they can choose to embrace the new knowledge, and thus grow, expand and ascend or try and squeeze it into old truths. This method will contaminate and negate the knowledge, so be open minded and prepared to learn and expand. Don't be stagnant and absolute in your thinking.

Another important realization I had as I progressed along this energy healing path, was that not only does the healer need to grow and expand energetically in order to become a bigger energy channel, they also need to cleanse themselves of their own baggage, traumas and negative beliefs. If they don't, as they grow energetically, so do their energetic traumas and scars. These can send them on their own fast-spinning downward spiral. Growing energetically is a double-edged sword.

Of course, this will also affect healings. You have to gain the knowledge and techniques and put them into practise, but you also have to clear yourself of your energetic baggage for your own benefit, as well as for your patients. These traumas and energetic entities will grow and torment you and affect your healings.

I realised this on my first trip to India. I was at the stage where I was growing energetically. My healings were amazing, and my intuition was sharp. I went there to live and study *Ayurveda* for two months with the experts. My focus was on learning and expanding. I was at Mumbai Airport at 3am in monsoon season, and lo and behold, the ATM kept rejecting my debit card. I had not a penny in my pocket, and my backpack was already tied on the top of the minibus. The driver was waiting for me to pay my fare and head off to Pune.

The minibuses leave when they're full, and this one was full with the engine revving. I was trying to convince the driver there was a problem with the ATM and that I could pay him when we got to the destination. He was reluctant and didn't know what to do, when a female passenger came up and said she'd pay my fare, and I could reimburse her when we got to the Ashram.

I was taken aback by this stranger's trust and generosity, and grateful for her offer. I followed her to the back of the bus, where we talked about the Ashram. That day I happened to be wearing maroon-coloured drawstring pants, and because this was the colour of the Ashram, she automatically assumed I was going there.

Well, this chance meeting changed my life forever. She spoke to me about this particular Ashram where the focus was on different types of meditations aimed at clearing all of the baggage that was dumped on you by your families, education systems, religions and cultures. She went on to say that it's good to shed these beliefs, as well as personal hurts and traumas, to become free to function from a place of personal choice through an increased level of awareness and empowerment.

This made perfect sense to me. I followed this girl to the Ashram and totally immersed myself in its meditations. When I'd completed my *Ayurvedic* course, I extended my visa and stayed at the Ashram, where I worked on clearing myself for the next three months. It was an enlightening time. So many realizations had come to light about how my character and beliefs had been shaped. There was realising and then releasing, which left me feeling happy and light and cleared my internal space, so I could be a bigger, cleaner channel for energy healing. This was a major revelation that the universe brought my way. I could have chosen not to investigate this Ashram and its offerings, and who knows where I'd be today? So, don't miss out. Receive your message.

There's another beautiful revelation I'd like to share, and this one also applies to everyone. It happened another time at the Ashram. I had decided to take *sannyas*, a ceremony where you pledge to yourself to seek the path of truth. It's an evening of celebration and high energy, and while we were jumping around and dancing, my then partner came up behind me, hugged and squeezed me and audibly inhaled my energy.

For a split second I had the thought, *That's right, suck up all of my energy.* Well, before I even completed the thought, I saw my heart chakra in front of my eyes, dazzling with bright colours and spinning clockwise. This indicated that it was activated. Not only was I ecstatic about clairvoyantly seeing my heart chakra, I was stunned with the message I'd received. Before I'd even finished my fallible thought, I was corrected. By sharing energy and love, you're not only giving but also receiving. You're activating your heart chakra, and the benefits are not only for your emotional wellbeing but for your physical body as well.

This revelation changed my life, and I never think twice about giving love to everything and everyone. Your gift bounces right back to you. Everyone on the spiritual journey receives their own revelations and realisations and has their truths adjusted. It's a beautiful process of growth. Be open to receiving and learning. You don't know who your teacher's going to be.

*From your own personal experiences, do you have a wholistic program that you follow or recommend?*

There are many great programs out there, and they all have something to offer. It depends on what the person needs and is looking for at that particular time. A wholistic program must include:

- organic, unprocessed food with minimal animal fats, like the Mediterranean diet

- a clean, fresh, healthy environment from which to breathe and exchange energy

- physical exercise, be it gentle or strenuous, which involves individual or group activities and sports, depending on the person's ability and preference

- meditation practices, including the traditional custom of silencing and emptying the mind, as well as various other meditations to connect and draw energy from the universe and then distribute it throughout the body to energise and heal

- positive thinking, higher emotions, love, compassion forgiveness and giving, and to remember that by doing good, you further activate your goodness, and therefore attract good energy to you.

The program I'm now using is based on the Ancient Greek healing system. I developed it whilst spending incredible summers on the Greek Islands. My healing experiences there led me to further research and apply the wisdom and principles of the Ancient Greeks, with amazing results.

**Can you further expand upon the Ancient Greek healing principles?**

Yes, let's get to know the Ancient Greeks.

▸ Ancient Greek medicine is the wholistic, documented healing system that current Western medicine is based upon.

▸ Ancient Greek medicine has many similarities in principles and practices with the *Ayurvedic* (Indian) and Chinese systems that were also developed simultaneously in different parts of the world.

▸ Hippocrates, a philosopher and physician in the fourth century B.C., first systemised and legitimised medicinal principles and practices. He systematically kept patients' records and methodically recorded scientific data and diagrams for later reference and study. This library of reference works constituted diseases and naturally occurring imbalances, war injuries and their treatment, as well as surgery and body anatomy diagrams.

▸ The Hippocratic Oath, by which he swore in physicians to maintain the higher ethics of their calling, is still used today with only the removal/adaptation of the part about prayers to gods and the forces of nature.

▸ The Ancient Greeks were the first to use the concept of hospitals, where the sick were removed from their homes and looked after in specialised places that were picked for their high-energy healing vibrations. They were always in the most pristine, natural settings, where physicians were on hand to observe, document and treat the various illnesses with an array of natural remedies.

▸ Even in the fourth century B.C., Hippocrates believed the mind and body are in unity, and to affect one is to affect the other.

- ▶ Hippocrates also believed that "All disease begins in the gut". Thus, extra attention is paid to the diet of the patients, as well as the use of local plants and herbs that had specialized constituents to help the body correct and harmonise certain malfunctions.

- ▶ The Ancient Greek medical system sought to harmonise the health of the individual with the Universal Life Force of Nature and the Cosmos. Their system was based on treating the four humours, or constitutions, of the individual in order to seek a balance, or homeostasis, with the opposing yet complementary forces of nature. They had a high respect for nature and using its forces to treat the body, mind and spirit.

- ▶ The Ancient Greeks also looked to the power of gods, or supernatural energy, for their healing, either directly or indirectly, and used rituals, prayers, hymns of praise and sacrifice to illicit the favours of their gods.

- ▶ The indirect method was through divine intervention, or the transmission of power by some agent such as a priest, healer or an object, by laying on of hands, touching or transferring this energy in some way.

- ▶ The direct method was following by directions the patient received in dreams and visions. Thus, the psychology and acceptance of these supernatural healings played an important part in the healing process.

- ▶ Belief was an integral part of the ancient healing arts. Connection with their gods, or an archetypal energy source through ritual and prayer, produced the activation of the healing powers within the patient. They understood the importance of stimulating the patient's own healing energies through the mind-body-spirit connection, for these miraculous transformations to take place.

**Do you have a retreat that encompasses these methods?**

Yes. My vision was to have the optimum location for a healing retreat. I was led to discover specific Greek Islands in the Aegean, where the energy vibration is high and clean. Places where half the healing occurs just by being there. I've developed a twenty-one day healing program, tailored to cater to small groups of people (a maximum of ten), that utilises all of the principles of the Ancient Greeks.

These retreats are specially created for people who've recovered from a major illness such as cancer, chronic fatigue, depression, an accident, or a traumatic divorce. They've survived, but they don't know where to turn for help to put their life back together again. It's a hands-on program, since most people have probably read enough, heard enough and know enough, and now is the time when they have to take action.

With careful and caring guidance by experienced healers, they're guided through the program, which includes morning energising exercises, yoga stretches, intense breathing techniques and an energising/ healing meditation, followed by a superfood breakfast. Group energy is important in healing. The total amount of energy generated by a group of seven people meditating together equals that of a hundred people meditating individually. There's also an evening meditation to help open the third eye and bring awareness and knowingness through dreams or visions to everyone's personal life situation.

It's been scientifically proven that it takes a minimum of twenty-one days to form a habit. This type of self-commitment is needed to recharge and regain your energy, youthfulness and joy. There's also a lot of fun to be had, such as swimming in crystal-clear waters, participating in cultural events, detoxing with mineral clay treatments on the beach, massaging for the physical body, and definitely energy healings using crystal wands to further speed the healing process or to move someone out of a healing crisis. Last, but not least, sharing this intense and special time in your life with a group of likeminded, positive, supportive people forms such lasting friendships and beautiful memories, most people don't want to leave.

More practical information about these retreats, including individual pre-retreat consultations to assess personal needs and to begin treatments and detoxing, as well as post-retreat follow-up sessions can be found on www.ancientgreekretreats.com

### What advice would you give to people who are learning about energy healing or are aspiring to become energy healers?

First of all, you must practise, practise, practise. No one becomes powerful and effective in energy healing by reading a book or even by doing a course. With these methods you get the fundamentals, but you also must put it into practice. This is the real learning. When you practise, you also observe what happens, how it feels, and how conditions change under different circumstances. You're learning and experimenting in different ways, and this learning is yours.

Once you've had this experience, no one can tell you it isn't so. You also learn to trust your gut instinct and develop your intuition. This knowingness is so important in energy healing, because you can't physically see what's there, but you can see it or feel it energetically. Hence, you develop your own style and discover what works best for you by using the principles you've already learnt.

I know from my own experience that it took me about two years of practising nearly every night with a buddy and healing family and friends, defining and refining my own guidance system, before I was confident to try it on strangers. Then, because I was confident in myself and my knowingness, my healings and consultations afterwards were really accurate. Also, people want you to share what you found and what's going on with them. They need to feel they're a part of the healing process, so don't keep it a mystery. Talk to them about it, and if appropriate, suggest what may have caused it.

Another final piece of advice is to drop the ego. You can't be a powerful healer if you're functioning from an egotistical place. You need to be a pure vessel, an open, receiving channel for the divine/universal energy to pass through. My most amazing healings were when I was at my lowest. For example, when my mother passed away, a week later I was an emotional and physical wreck, and I had to do an emergency healing on a patient, because his kidney creatinine levels were so high that he was going to be put on dialysis the next day if they were the same in the morning's blood test. Even in my wrecked state I couldn't refuse to treat him, so I totally gave in to source and being an energy channel. I can honestly say there wasn't a shred of ego in me. Well, the morning tests showed his creatinine levels were back to normal. How amazing is that?

When I sense ego in a healer, I know their healing is going to be limited.

### Do you have any final thoughts?

My final word on energy healing is that it's no mystery. It's part of the natural world. The universality of energy just needs to be recognised. Once there's an understanding of how everyone is made up of the same light particles and that energy isn't static but changes and moves according to emotions, environment and health, a person can learn to move it, clear it and manipulate it to achieve the desired results.

But learning and comprehending the power of energy are just the first steps to becoming an energy healer. Good fundamentals and a sound proven tradition is a good place to start, but to be an energy healer it's important to have heart and work from a place of love, connect with the universal source and put loving intention into each and every healing.

The final ingredients are passion and commitment. A good energy healer should be open and intuitive, and then practise, fine tune and evolve this intuition. Energy healers must cleanse themselves of their own traumas, untruths and baggage that may become obstacles to becoming a large, clean vessel for the energy to channel through. Once the path is cleared, there's no limit to the magic that can be created.

 To discover more about how Catherine can help you *Elevate Your Health*, visit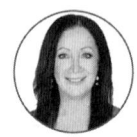

www.elevate-books.com/health

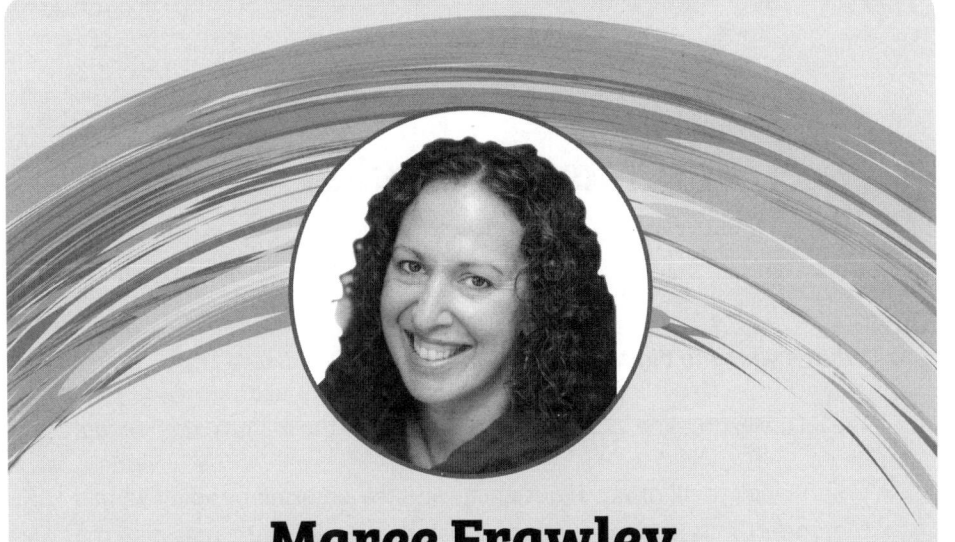

# **Maree Frawley**

## Rejuvenate Your Purpose

Maree Frawley is an expert in rejuvenation of the physical and emotional body. She believes every person can live an inspired life, full of vitality and a balance of support and challenge. She has taught more than 18,000 group fitness sessions, facilitated the conditioning and performance of elite athletes, conducted more than 11,000 sessions of personal training, helped improve the health of expecting mothers, and assisted those with chronic pain or those in the process of reclaiming their health and fitness.

As a rejuvenation specialist, Maree utilises, superior implementation of biomechanics, high-performance coaching, mindset techniques, yoga, mindfulness and meditation.

As a mum of twins and a business owner/manager, she understands the necessity of having optimal health to thrive and live with inspired purpose. Maree is no stranger to pain and adversity. Her teachings, combined with her experiences, have assisted her in helping thousands of clients achieve inspired vitality

Maree provides simple pathways for mindfulness and outstanding nurturing support. She helps those in need find clarity amid the confusion of deciphering the best options for personal vitality, including nutrition, exercise, emotional management and mindset.

# Maree Frawley

## Rejuvenate Your Purpose

### What's your the biggest life lesson?

I avoid the expression, *Don't quit* and instead use the mantra, *Keep Going*!

When I look at all of my experiences and the amazing people I've had the opportunity to work with, I realise there's a phrase that gets me through the good and challenging days. It's, *Yes, you can!*

Although I've read statements and been told from an early age that every day is a precious gift, I think it's through health challenges, loss of loved ones and overcoming adversity that I've been able to live as though every day is the most precious gift and amazing opportunity to bring love and balance into my life, as well as the lives of others. My children and partner certainly help.

A kind word, a smile, a shared giggle, a hug, a moment of relaxation or a quality moment when someone needs it, can save a life. I've seen it. I've felt it.

When times are tough, keep going. What if you were next to receive your rewards or achieve your goal, and then you hopped out of line because it was taking too long? You wind up at the back of the line again. Instead of giving up, hang in there. Keep doing one percent more every day.

### What does love mean to you?

Until the last few years, my understanding of love was that it a feeling you simply had towards another person, and maybe on a good day towards yourself.

 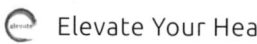

But through my investigation of philosophy, religions and attending seminars, especially those by Dr John Demartini and Ben Harvey, my awareness of love as a vibration and state of being allowed me to understand how it can heal and help a person stay balanced and content. Being alive, living your magnificence, and helping people to live their magnificence, is part of this state of being. It brings you into the present moment where there's clarity and a pure vibration of healing, connection and flowing energy.

### If you were speaking to your younger self, what advice would you give?

In the midst of an emotionally challenging time, I came across a picture of a rodeo rider nearly being bucked off his horse, but he was still holding on. The caption read, *I know God wouldn't give me anything I couldn't handle, I just wish I wasn't trusted so much.* There's also the same quote on a picture with Mother Theresa. This phrase has been a pillar of inspiration for me.

And this is where I would start my advice:

You're only given lessons you can handle, so embrace the experiences and see the perfect balance of every situation. Understand you're receiving the lessons you need in order to become the person you're destined to be.

There's a suburban folklore story about making the most of your circumstances. It involves a carrot, coffee and boiling water. When the water boils for a long period of time, will you let it whither and weaken you like the carrot, allow it to make you hard in the middle like a boiled egg, or will you own the situation and transform the water, like the coffee granules do?

Everyone has their own talent and calling. It's when you open your heart to the grand plan and align yourself with it, that everything will fall into place as it's meant to. Continue to transform your experiences into the understanding of wisdom that will help you live your extraordinary life.

Don't sweat the small stuff, but make sure you do the little things that make the most extraordinary difference to yourself and others.

Above all, hang in there while you're able and alive. You're a child of the universe and have every given blessing to live your own magnificence.

With your pursuit and experience of knowledge, there comes responsibility to care for the knowledge, educate others and participate in human evolution. One lone voice can inspire a million to expand their mind. Dare to be the most amazing version of you.

### How would you like to be remembered?

As a balanced, wise and peaceful mother, wife, sister, daughter and friend who inspired people to continue their journey towards their goals and life purpose, had a joyous sense of humour and kept people laughing when they didn't think it was possible. As someone who helped people find a state of balance when all hope was lost, their breath in times they could only find pain and their vibration of love where they once experienced fear and anxiety.

### What is the one message you wish to share with the world?

What matters is this moment, right now. Change your thoughts, and you change your life. You're extraordinary, and you're able to live the life, achieve the goals and feel the way you wish to.

Life has seasons, and each one will have extremes, yet at the same time absolute balance. Adapt, modify and move with the current challenges and joys. This season will pass, and you will be a wiser and more empowered version of yourself. Begin with awareness of your breath and understand the simplicity of getting your brain to focus and be calm. Awareness of the breath will then flow to body awareness, mind awareness and better clarity throughout the day.

**What's the worst thing that's ever happened to you, and how did you overcome it?**

Having spent a lot of time balancing out and appreciating the lessons of the bigger life events that would fit into this category, I do feel that all of the challenges I've faced have been priceless gifts.

Just before my twenty-first birthday, I was in a reasonably significant car accident. It happened after I completed my commerce degree via correspondence at the University of New England.

I experienced reasonably significant challenges post car accident. It gave me a great gift: the journey and discovery of managing a great deal of back and neck pain. Even so, I was driven to return to my active lifestyle, and I pushed hard to get back to teaching group fitness classes, doing personal training and pursuing my own fitness training.

I know there are people who aren't yet in a place where they can understand how chronic pain is a gift. For about ten years I was nowhere near this understanding, even when I was working with people who experienced far worse injury than I ever did. The day-in and day-out struggle is endless, and the fog of whether it's ever going to end clouds everything, like relationships, career and business. Everything.

I can honestly say that the natural birth of my twins didn't compare to the emotional and physical challenges I experienced during the periods of debilitating back pain. There were three significant episodes to this point in my life where for extended periods I was not able to walk. Since I lived a perceivably fit and healthy lifestyle, I realised people had a hard time understanding what was going on. Comments were made in my fitness, Pilates and yoga classes about how they thought I would be more flexible, and it left me with the belief system that I must soldier on, because no one would understand.

Yet the gifts in these situations more than equalled the challenges. My immersion into biomechanics and the ability to inspire, nurture, empathise and guide people through their physical and emotional rejuvenation, has helped me bring out the best in my clients and assist me every day to bring the best out in myself.

It took seventeen years of rehabilitation, but I got my hip to release. I'm stronger and more stable, physically and emotionally, than I've ever been before. All of the tools and experiences now benefit my clients.

### Have you had any aha moments that changed everything for you?

Becoming a mum. The way the world looks pre and post baby, is so incredibly different. More than ever, I understand the importance of legacy and the world we're leaving for our children and future generations.

I thought I was pretty strong carrying the twins to thirty-nine weeks, teaching high-impact aerobics up until thirty-six weeks, and yoga until the night before the babies were born, and figured most of the challenges were behind me. I was wrong.

While in the hospital, I'd been having trouble with my body temperature, so a nurse laid a jacket over me. I'd barely slept in five days. Although the angels, aka the nurses of the NICU, and almost all of the midwives were amazing, on day five a midwife came into my hospital room, opened the curtain and yelled at me, "You've suffocated one of your babies!" I sat up, and my heart raced as I burst into tears. I was disoriented and wondering what had happened, but my partner, Kevin, was absolutely irate and took care of the situation.

There was no apology or clarification, just the midwife's explanation that she saw my jacket beside me and thought I was on top of a baby. It seems surreal and weird, but it was a reminder of the way the world works and how people can perceive the same moment in time so incredibly differently.

So what was the aha moment?

This event empowered me to speak up and speak out. I muscled up and became the mother lion. I realised I had to take responsibility for myself, my partner and my babies and say that what happened was insane and so far from okay. It was a moment that took me quite a few years to balance out, but the immediate lesson I learned about how to speak up, protect and nurture carries into how I instruct yoga and address large groups. I appreciate the empowerment and awareness to use my voice regardless of the environment and situation.

Meeting Kevin and finding our way into a high-functioning relationship was another amazing aha moment. During my pregnancy with the twins, he fractured his femur, so after the babies were born I realised it was necessary and okay to ask for and accept help.

On a business level, the asking for help or accessing of leverage is necessary from staff and consultants and has been a straightforward process that overcame the idea of being too proud. It's okay to put your hand up. It's brilliant to go do a course or attend a seminar.

I've learnt that just as I love supporting and being there for others, people want to do the same for me. This goes for you as well. Allow others to use their talents in reciprocation. It's the law of balance.

### What decisions have made a difference in your life?

Persisting with yoga and becoming a yoga instructor was an important decision.

My family works hard, so it's no surprise that in my mid-twenties I had a ridiculous routine of constantly doing something. I had no idea how to just be. My normal day started at 4:30 a.m. I'd teach fitness classes, do corporate work, train people and study at night. I averaged two-three hours of sleep per night. I was extremely fit, in chronic pain, had poor nutrition and was in constant adrenal overload. It was no surprise when I crashed out and was forced to find a path of balance.

When I first started yoga, I had no understanding of it and truly resented being in the classes, but over a few months I continued trying different styles until I found a pathway that suited me, and I've stuck with it and reaped the rewards ever since.

Yoga may not be for every person, but a pathway for finding balance is essential. I think every decision is an evolution of spirit, even on the most basic level of embracing responsibility rather than resenting it, and has been fundamental to my achievements.

### What's the best thing that's ever happened to you and why?

Being part of my beautiful family and becoming a mother to our beautiful twins is the biggest and most continuous daily transforming experience I've had.

They've already heard some of the pep talks I've given to athletes. Before the age of five, my children have sat though seminars and listened to them when we're driving in the car. They've been in the yoga room since they were born and understand the need for taking time to refocus.

They challenge and demand me to look deep within for what I need to learn in order to help and inspire them to live their own magnificence, while I live mine.

### What is your big WHY?

My loving partner, Kevin, and my beautiful children, Katea and Kaiyu. Finding balance is a gift I love to share with all I meet.

**How are you currently making a difference in people's lives?**

With my chiropractic and yoga health centre, Port Stephens Chiropractic and Yoga. My partner is a chiropractor, and I run a variety of programs in therapeutic yoga that's gentle and specific for the needs of the class. The yoga I teach is a fusion of my skill set that is harmonious to the philosophy and asana work of yoga.

I do rejuvenation consultations for people wanting musculoskeletal balance, pain management and hormonal and emotional balance. I also do rejuvenation movement sessions, which are a combination of body work, activation, release and movement.

I run retreat days and host workshops in schools and the corporate environment to inspire people to break their monotony and live the life they dream of through learning to breathe optimally, understanding their unique bio-individuality and focusing.

**What inspires you, and what are you passionate about?**

I'm inspired by transformation. I love seeing people achieve what they could only dream about. I love the preparation and pathway that's experienced way before the goal is ticked or the game is won.

I'm passionate about:

- walking people down the pathway of reducing their body weight

- pulling together a rugby club that had been full of turmoil and racism to win a grand final

- helping people crippled by emotional limitation to set goals and transform into a self-believer

- assisting the fragile in rebuilding foundations and moving into a strong place

- facilitating those debilitated by pain and dysfunction to balance out and reclaim vitality

- getting people to sparkle with inspiration and self fulfilment

**With your experience, what's the biggest tip you could give people?**

Be consistent!

If you haven't exercised for a while, just do one percent more than you did yesterday. The next day do another percent. In a year's time you will be further ahead than if you exert yourself too much and wind up getting sick and injured and out of commission for weeks at a time.

Maintain balance and remember to go for your challenges, but be your best friend and nurture yourself. The smallest, consistent improvements over time lead to a long, consistent leap forward.

Every day is a gift, so be loving to yourself, and make time to breathe and be mindful.

**What can someone do right now to change their life?**

While you're reading this, lengthen your spine and take a couple of balanced, easy and relaxed breaths.

**What's the biggest mistake people make in the area of reclaiming their fitness and health?**

When you're fit and healthy, you can build on and build up, because you've given yourself a firm foundation. Also, it's important to understand that being fit doesn't always go hand in hand with being healthy. There are a lot of reasonably fit people who still carry injuries, weight and nutritional habits that lead them in the opposite direction of health gains.

When you have limitations, injuries, time constraints and a strategy of pushing too hard and feeling the pain, it will lead you down a path of adrenal overload and chronic injury.

In the late nineties I presented workshops regarding chemistry and hormones and the role of the stress cycle in weight gain and catabolic affects on the body. There needs to be a balance. Whenever there's an adrenal response, the body requires more nurturing.

People need to consider their unique bio-individuality, their history and their goals, and take action accordingly. They need to choose the appropriate activities and/or trainers.

I have a twenty-year history of training hard, which I now choose not to do. This is a decision I still grapple with. However, the more moderate I am, the more I notice my overall quality of life is better. I see this in my clients as well.

My advice for a person with back pain or an injury is to start small and progress.

The fundamentals of a hundred-metre sprint are completely different from a marathon. This is why it's important to define what role you want exercise and fitness to play in your life and choose activities accordingly.

The exercise and weight loss industries have always had a fad component. That's what keeps the mass population involved. It's okay to participate in these fads if they have a positive outcome on your body and emotions, as enjoyment and self-belief are crucial.

Even small changes make the biggest difference. Here are some examples:

▶ Learn how to breathe correctly.

▶ Discover how to activate inactive muscles.

▶ Stretch short, tight muscles and stabilise long, weak muscles.

▶ Fuel your body for nutrition, not just weight loss.

▶ Drink good-quality water.

▶ Practice appreciation and mindfulness.

▶ Be consistent.

### What's your most inspiring client story?

Firstly, I do want to say I've loved and want to thank everyone I've worked with, and will work with in the future. The inspirations pile is high, because I've dealt with people overcoming physical challenges, but one in particular stands out.

I had a phone call from the daughter of a ninety-one year old man who wanted me to train him. She asked me to go around to his house to see if he liked me. This made me laugh already.

When I arrived at his house, this barely five feet tall, heavily hunched over man came out to greet me. He walked slowly, and the first question he asked me in his thick accent was, "Do you believe in Him?" He pointed to the sky. "Because Him and me, we don't get along." In an era of political correctness, this was an unusual question, and my tactic of remaining silent seemed to be a sufficient answer.

At this first meeting, I was humbled, inspired and driven to help him achieve his goal.

This dear client, now departed from this world, was Dr Bernard Ingram, a Jewish survivor of the Holocaust. He'd come to Australia not able to speak a word of English. He lost his identity, had to do his medical degree a few times over and supported the Newcastle community with amazing medical service. Over a period of six months he was able to balance on one leg and reach behind his head, so he no longer needed live-in care, as he could shower and dress himself again.

We spent two years together for two hours per week. He was a champion for life and gave me great insight. We joked about training for the Olympics for the sport of Judo, and he reminded me of the importance of exercising your brain. Every day he completed the nine-letter word brain teaser out of the newspaper and challenged me to do the same. He spoke six languages and would often question whether English was my first language.

He referred to himself as a normal man, but he was the epitome of resilience and was aligned to the philosophy of just hanging in there. He helped me understand the bigger picture of fitness and wellbeing, as well as the importance of etiquette and manners, and how in any given situation I needed to do what I could, because everything else would take care of itself. He taught me that no matter how small your effort, to keep going.

### What is your approach to your rejuvenation and inspiration?

By nature, our world values complexity, but the system to rejuvenation is simple:

▸ Get clear on the quality of life you're striving for.

▸ Work on your mindset and self-belief

▸ Design the system of nutrition and exercise needed for your bio-individuality.

▸ Do one percent more than you did the day before when making any changes.

- Focus daily on mindset.

- Learn how to breathe for balance, core strength and energy. The most established yogis and athletes, to people who feel broken, need to practice their breathing technique

- Eat for nutrition and energy.

- Exercise for vitality, energy and lifestyle improvements.

- Be consistent.

**What courses have you taken that enabled you to get started or build your business?**

I wear many hats. Part of my journey has been to embrace the diversity and enjoy the responsibility of the numerous components of my business.

From managing our chiropractic and yoga centre, teaching yoga and hosting retreat days, corporate and school workshops, property management, domestic goddess duties and being a loving partner and mother, the courses for success have been numerous.

- Bachelor of Commerce, University of New England Studies, via correspondence

- Masters Business Administration, UNE, via correspondence

- Cert III in Fitness Group Fitness/Gym Instruction/Aqua Instruction. Includes certification in Les Mill's programs, Master Trainer in fit ball techniques and advanced lifting techniques

  - Cert IV in Fitness Personal Training/Specific Populations

  - Advanced Diploma Yoga RYTA 500

- Pilates certified

- Certificate IV Training and Assessment

- Certificate IV in Business

- Steve McKnight's Property Apprenticeship (property investing)

- Steve McKnight Born to Be Financially Free mentoring program

- Authentic Education PHD: Programs for Heart-Centered Difference-Makers

- John Demartini Breakthrough seminar

Plus many, many more.

### What's the best way people can achieve a good life-work balance?

This is something I lacked for the best part of seventeen years. I worked seven days a week and gave every ounce of energy to my work.

It was during a conversation with a client that it occurred to me I was giving the best part of my energy to my clients, and sometimes perfect strangers, and I started to realise that those I hold dearest should be the ones to see and be with the best of me.

My dear partner, Kevin, has taught me a great deal about having a good work-life balance. When we started our business together and were living on the work premises, it was important to establish a space for family and a space for work. Even just little considerations we developed over time, such as talking about work in the kitchen and not our bedroom, was a great choice for balancing our relationship.

The challenge of maintaining a healthy work-life balance for us was determined by the high value we placed on family and ensuring we invested the time to stay strong and thrive. Having a family day and establishing a commitment to enjoying the holiday lifestyle of the beautiful town we live in are all part of the ability to manage a healthy life-work balance. We're moving into organic farming, so there's a whole new level of balance required to ensure our health and wellbeing, as well as growing together as a family and as a couple.

### Why is mindset important?

I'd always read sayings such as, *Change your thoughts, and you can change your life*, but I didn't realise how powerful this was until I added a daily discipline to my thinking.

How much energy and time did I lose due to thinking beyond the moment and about issues that have a negative emotional charge? This is in contrast to living with a balanced mind, in order to stabilise emotional charges and maintain personal power.

For years I helped people break through pain and physical limitations, as well as dealing with my own, but a whole new world opened up when I changed my mindset about other areas of my life, including relationships and finances.

Everyone has challenges. Another gift I was given was during a time when I developed vocal nodules. It happened post car accident, due to my change of posture and strain whilst instructing. I was advised to have three months of silence to enhance healing rather than have surgery. Whispering is poison to vocal chords, so I had three months of writing notes and simply being silent. It was no wonder my relationship ended, since my boyfriend was unable to read.

The voices in my head were usually drowned out by banter and business, so I had to confront all of the poison. This is when I learnt the power of deeply listening to myself and others. I had the opportunity to apply mindset to healing and to making the most of the cards life had dealt me.

### How does someone keep inspired on a daily basis?

▶ Have gratitude.

▶ Set a daily intention.

▶ See the movie of your day.

▶ Work toward the script of your life.

▶ Maintain balance.

▶ Do what's aligned to your life purpose.

▶ Laugh!

▶ Do what bring you joy.

I do lose balance, and I have a tool box that consists of what I learned from Demartini and Ben Harvey's Authentic Education, to bring me back into balance.

### What are some tools or strategies you'd recommend for maintaining balance?

It's okay to push hard, but at some point you deliberately need to swing the pendulum back to nurturing yourself, otherwise your body and emotions will take you there through injury, illness, setback or a plateau.

When you look at nature, you can see it has periods of challenge and long periods of recovery. Life, technology, poor rest, nutrient-lacking food and questionable water quality are overloading your body with toxicity. You need to take time to nurture and rebalance.

Maybe you're collapsing or completely overloaded. Then there are parents who are aware their child can't sit still and doesn't know how to relax but don't know what to do about it. The good news is that anyone can learn skills to balance out their life.

My life used to be manic. My definition of balance with exercise was to throw in some low-impact aerobics or water training. It didn't cross my mind to go further into the spectrum of mindfulness. Life is a journey, and I need to tell my fellow manic personalities to ease themselves into mindfulness. Try breathing techniques and mindful movement. Maybe some *tai chi*, *chi gung* or standing on the beach and letting your feet sink into the sand as the water goes out.

Truly appreciate there's no right or wrong. It's just a process of bringing balance into your life. Many people experiencing yoga for the first time have challenges just giving themselves permission to do less and simply be. But once they remove the self and their perceived expectations, they love the feeling of being centred, aware and in a state of appreciation.

### Do you have a coach or mentor or someone to motivate you?

I have many.

My partner, Kevin Schwager. He will do whatever he can to improve the lives of everyone around him. He's the strongest spirit I've ever met.

My twins. They make me look within and discover how I can be better in all areas of my life.

Steve McKnight. When I needed a pathway of knowledge to move our family forward, it wasn't just his property apprenticeship, but his program of Born to be Financially Free that allowed me to discover the depth of humanity and brilliance of his integrity. To run a program at no cost but include standards that if not met, meant self-elimination from the program, highlighted the importance of consistency. Over a two-year period, there were less than twenty people left from 250. Every trip to Melbourne was worth it, and my family, as well as all of the people we continue to help, have benefited from his influence in our lives.

Ben Harvey and Authentic Education. The awesomeness of this man's knowledge and ability to communicate is a gift I truly treasure. His tools, systems and programs have improved my life in all areas.

Dallas Rosekelly, my first boss and lifelong friend. He's always helped me overcome my fear of living the life I appreciate now.

Gerry Gourley, my amazing balance. He helped me understand the value of establishing some limits and boundaries. He was part of the process of me moving beyond pain and survival to living my life in *thrival*.

Pretty much every client who gives me the opportunity to work with them in some way has become a mentor, as I look within to help guide and support them to their goals.

### Is meditation or mindfulness something everyone should practice?

I think it's important to appreciate the scope of meditation practices that are out there and for each individual to give themselves time to explore how to best bring themselves into a focused mind and be present in the moment.

So yes, I think everyone should practice mindfulness and meditation, but in the form that's best for them.

During my first yoga class, I felt expectations from the people around me, as well as the instructor. Physically, my pain was excruciating. I cramped in the most simple kneeling posture variation. Emotionally, I wanted to be anywhere other than in the session. So if a person is challenged by sitting still, maybe a more active yoga session with some mediation at the end or simply walking along the beach may be a starting point to build upon.

***What are your tips for getting through a difficult time in life?***

When times are tough, life is polishing and preparing you for the next round of opportunities that will allow you to live life to the fullest and find your purpose. Instead of giving up, hang in there. Keep doing one percent more every day!

 To discover more about how Maree can help you *Elevate Your Health*, visit

www.elevate-books.com/health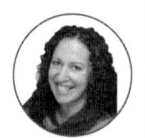

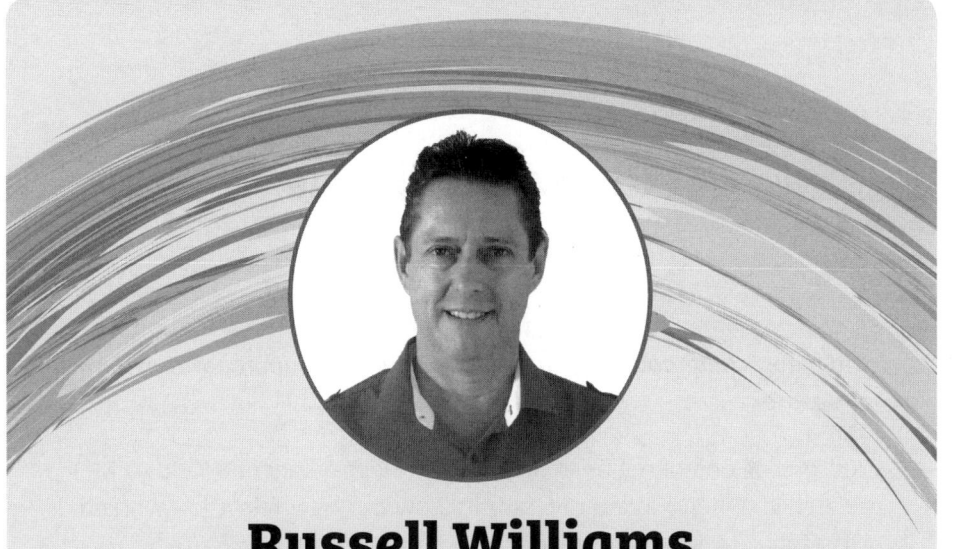

# Russell Williams

## The Invisible Enemy

Russell started his career as a laboratory technician in the pharmaceutical industry in England before completing an Honours degree in Environmental Studies at Sunderland University in 1984.

Since moving to Australia in 1988, Russell has worked at the National Occupational Health and Safety Commission, NSW State Pollution Control Commission, has filled various scientific roles and undertaken a number of housing management and advisory positions.

Due to his interest in the impact of urban living, specifically the health impacts of living in the modern-built environment, Russell is now the Director of Building Harmony Pty., a Building Biology consultancy where he assists homeowners, renters and small businesses. The services he provides include assessment of the health impacts of indoor air quality issues, including those produced by volatile organic compounds (chemicals) in building materials and household products, allergens in and around the home and electromagnetic field issues. He offers practical solutions to the issues he encounters.

# Russell Williams

## The Invisible Enemy

**Did your childhood play a role in your passion regarding EMF exposure?**

Yes. I recall one of my first exposures to Electromagnetic Fields (EMF) as a child, when I asked my parents how our new television worked. I'd started to sit close to get the whole at-the-movies effect. They explained what they knew, which is that the pictures came out through radio waves and likened it to the technology they'd used decades earlier. "You mean something I can't see is showing me the picture?" I asked. "Yes" was the only answer I got. My parents were average people of their day, not scientists. Later, I learnt these invisible waves were all around and even passed through people. I have since discovered they're coming from an increasing number of sources. There's little or no respite, as they seem to be everywhere you go.

**Are people today safe inside their home?**

It's a common belief that people spend much of their time at home, either awake or asleep. It's their castle, their refuge from the stress and struggles of the outside world. It's the place where the whole family enjoys their time together and feels safe.

I need to dispel that myth, because there's no assurance you're safe inside your home.

There's an unseen enemy that can sneak up on you without you even knowing it. EMFs are produced by appliances, recreational consoles and any other devices that use an electrical current. As Lyn Mclean, author and educator says, "It's invisible and inaudible; you can't smell, taste or touch it."

Elevate Your Health

Though few people are aware of the existence of EMF, trust me, it's out there. However, there's no need to be paranoid. You just need to know what to do to protect yourself, as it can have an effect on your health.

Those particularly susceptible to it are babies, growing children and pregnant women. But have no fear, greater safety comes with increased awareness, so you can make informed choices. Everyone can become a little safer by gaining a little knowledge.

The world has become reliant on the benefits electricity brings, but you also need to consider its risks. Wherever possible, you should put distance between yourself and a source of EMF. Its strength is inversely proportionate to the distance from it. Put simply, for each doubling of the distance, you reduce the field strength to a quarter of what it was.

### What got you interested in EMF?

EMFs first came to my attention while I was studying for my environmental studies degree about thirty years ago and then later when I worked in occupational health and safety. At that stage, EMF in the home environment was not considered a serious issue but more of an occupational exposure problem.

However, as everyone now uses more and more electrical devices, and at a younger age than ever before, EMF exposure in the home is a major concern. The use of technology has become more widespread, and there are few who aren't exposed to it. The most unfortunate consequence is the lack of awareness of its existence and the broad range of impacts it potentially has on the human body.

### Where is EMF found?

Wherever electric current flows through a wire or cable, there's an electromagnetic field. Physicists always associate the presence of the two together, like a knife is to a fork.

As electromagnetic fields are everywhere, they interact with the human physiology on a number of levels. Even the blood circulating from the heart is electrically charged and produces a measurable magnetic field. The earth itself has a magnetic field. But just because it's everywhere doesn't make it harmless when you're exposed to it at high levels, or even at low levels for an extended period. Some people are sensitive to electromagnetic fields and are affected by low field strengths.

EMF is measured in units called Tesla or Gauss. Tesla is an SI unit for electromagnetism, like metre or foot is to distance. Tesla is used in Australia and European countries, while a Gauss is a scale of measurement adopted in the USA. As field strengths are often small, they're measured in either milliGauss (mG, or a thousandth of a Gauss) or a microTesla (a millionth of a Tesla). An mG is equal to 0.1 microTesla. I will be referring to both.

The main emitters of EMF in the home are everyday devices such as your electric cooker, hot water service, TV, hairdryers, computer, Wi-Fi, and microwave (see table below). But given that Wi-Fi communication is often on continuously in most homes, I consider that to be of growing concern.

The US Environmental Protection Agency (EPA) has provided recommended safety levels of 0.5mG-2.5 mG for certain appliances. But these should be considered in the context of scientific recommendations outlined in the BioInitiative Report, which is set at 1mG and the more conservative Building Biology recommendation of 0.2mG. As the US EPA appliance list is not large, I've supplemented it with information sourced from the Australian Radiation Authority (ARPANSA).

| Source | Up to 4 inches away (10 cm) (US EPA) mG | At 3 feet (US EPA) (1metre) mG | ARPANSA[1] (at normal operating distance) mG |
|---|---|---|---|
| Blender | 50-220 | 0.3-3 | - |
| Clothes washer | 8-200 | 0.1-4 | - |
| Coffee maker | 6-29 | 0.1 | - |
| Computer | 4-20 | 2-5 | 2-20 |
| Fluorescent Lamp | 400-4000 | 0.1-5 | - |
| Hair Dryer | 60-20,000 | 0.1-6 | 10-70 |
| Microwave oven | 100-500 | 1-25 | - |
| Television | 5-100 | 0.1-6 | 0.2-2 |
| Vacuum Cleaner | 230-1,300 | 3-40 | - |
| Electric Stove | - | - | 2-30 |
| Refrigerator | - | - | 2-5 |
| Electric kettle | - | - | 2-10 |
| Electric blanket | | | 5-30 |
| Toaster | - | - | 2-10 |
| Pedestal fan | - | - | 0.2-2 |

1. Australian Radiation Protection and Nuclear Safety Agency

As you can see, distancing yourself from appliances is a good idea. While for some devices it isn't practical, like with hairdryers, vacuum and computers, try using them during daylight hours due to the impact of EMF on melatonin, which plays a protective role in the body.

## What is electromagnetic hypersensitivity (EHS)?

The BioInitiative Working Group[2] considers electromagnetic hypersensitivity as a neurological syndrome that's an emerging health problem. There are a range of symptoms reported, and they can arise at much lower EMF levels than the adopted safety guidelines.

EHS Symptoms can include:

- cognitive dysfunction (poor memory and problem-solving)
- balance challenges (vertigo)
- facial flushing
- poor concentration
- dizziness
- skin rash
- chest pressure
- rapid heart rate
- depression
- anxiety
- sleeplessness
- body aches
- headaches
- tinnitus
- symptoms consistent with chronic fatigue and fibromyalgia.

2. The BioInitiative Working Group is an independent group of 29 scientists who have reviewed the growing evidence on the effects of EMF exposure and produced a set of periodic reports on their findings. It presents a solid scientific and public health policy assessment that is evidence--based.

If you have one or more of these symptoms that can't be explained as a symptom of a diagnosed illness or pharmaceutical side effect, you need to investigate whether EMF in your environment could be the cause. A growing number of people are becoming highly sensitive to EMF.

## What do regulators say?

Each country has its own set of regulators for radiation safety. However, most exposure standards appear to be based on international guidelines set by the World Health Organisation's International Agency for Research into Cancer (IARC).

These guidelines are often criticised, as they're set at such a high EMF level that was based on inducing thermal effects in human tissue. Other effects can manifest a while before the exposure standard is reached, and unless you're knowledgeable about the situation, you won't know the level of exposure you've experienced.

It's always easy to be critical in hindsight. A useful example is the earlier practice in the 1930s to 1950s of the permitted use of radioactivity on the population. Women had unwanted hair removed using x-rays, psychiatric patients were treated with radium and small children were exposed to x-rays in shoe shops as a means to accurately check the fit of a shoe. While these practices are considered cringe-worthy now, they were as acceptable as the use of a hair dryer, mobile phone or Wi-Fi are these days. Perhaps the current applications of technology might get the same reaction from people in twenty or thirty years.

As Dr Devra Davis, an epidemiologist and founding director of the Center for Environmental Oncology, puts it, "We are in the middle of a global experiment but one without a control group."

### What do the scientists say?

Science has not been able to provide the unequivocal evidence policymakers and regulators appear to need for them to adequately protect the public. Manufacturers of mobile phones keep changing the radiofrequencies, making it difficult for scientists to study exposure over an extended period.

Manufacturers seem to only care about the bottom line and not how harmful the devices they sell can be in the long term. For instance, peer-reviewed scientific research is usually disputed by industry-sponsored research. It muddies the waters, because it comes up with results that either appear inconclusive or cast doubt on properly conducted scientific research. You may recall that the same tactic was used by the tobacco lobby. In the face of growing scientific evidence and bad publicity, they used their own research and combined it with confounding media statements. And you know how that turned out, don't you?

Regulators seem to be taking a wait-and-see approach until *good* science tips the scales.

I would like to end with a message from Professor David Carpenter, M.D. Dr Carpenter is the Director of the Institute for Health and the Environment, School of Public Health, University of Albany, USA.

*"Studies of people have shown that both ELF and RF exposures result in an increased risk of cancer, and that this occurs at intensities that are too low to cause tissue heating. Unfortunately, all of our exposure standards are based on the false assumption that there are no hazardous effects at intensities that do not cause tissue heating. Based on the existing science, many public health experts believe it is possible we will face an epidemic of cancers in the future, resulting from uncontrolled use of cell phones and increased population exposure to Wi-Fi and other wireless devices. Thus it is important that all of us, and*

*especially children, restrict our use of cell phones, limit exposure to background levels of Wi-Fi, and that government and industry discover ways in which to allow use of wireless devices without such elevated risk of serious disease. We need to educate decision-makers that 'business as usual' is unacceptable. The importance of this public health issue cannot be underestimated."*

### What are other countries doing to protect their population?

While the regulators aren't on board yet, the scientific evidence is continuing to mount.

A number of countries have accepted that "presumption of innocence" doesn't work as a public health policy (Blank, 2014). Consequently, they've acted to protect their populations by using the precautionary principle[3] to limit exposure and protect vulnerable groups such as young children and pregnant women. Others are waiting to see if regulators are going to make more unambiguous statements about the risks.

Some countries have acted on the precautionary principle. For instance in Brussels, Belgium They established a precautionary limit for 900Hz mobile phone base stations, which is one-fourteenth that of the International commission on Non-Ionising Radiation Protection (ICNIRP) guidelines. Canada responded to a 2010 report on Wi-Fi by removing it from some schools.

Australia doggedly follows the ICNIRP guidelines, meaning we're falling behind the international community in acting to protect its population.

3. The Precautionary Principle is defined as: 'When human activities may lead to morally unacceptable harm that is scientifically plausible but uncertain, actions shall be taken to avoid or diminish that harm. Morally unacceptable harm refers to harm to humans or the environment that is – threatening to human life or health, or – serious and effectively irreversible, or – inequitable to present or future generations, or --imposed without adequate consideration of the human rights of those affected. Actions are interventions that are undertaken before harm occurs that seek to avoid or diminish the harm. ' The United Nations Educational, Scientific and Cultural Organization (UNESCO) – 2005 World Commission on the Ethics of Scientific Knowledge and Technology

In 2010, the Environment and Health Committee of the Israeli Parliament recommended the government prevent exposure of students to electromagnetic fields, due to concerns about Wi-Fi. In 2011, the Council of Europe Committee on the Environment, Agriculture and Local Regional Affairs, recommended to its member nations that mobile phones, DECT phones, Wi-Fi and WLAN systems be banned from classrooms.

There have been many failures to use the precautionary principle. Instead, dangerous products and materials have continued to be used for extended periods after health effects began to be known, such as DDT, asbestos and Thalidomide.

### What are the risks of EMF to a person's health?

There are health effects attributed to exposure to extremely low frequency electromagnetic fields (ELF) associated with power generation, electrical wiring and household electrical appliances.

While these numbers seem scary, you need to know the risks in order to protect yourself. Please know many exposures are avoidable if you take the proper precautions.

- A panel of eminent scientists have stated unequivocally in the BioInitiative report of 2012, *There is little doubt that exposure to ELF causes childhood leukaemia.*

- The increased risk for childhood leukaemia starts at levels almost a thousand times below the safety standard and doubles for young boys at only 1.4 mG and above (Green et al, 1999). IARC has classified magnetic fields of above 4 mG as possibly carcinogenic.

- Strong evidence exists that long-term exposure to ELF, as well as EMF's impact on melatonin, are linked to the risk of Alzheimer's disease. ELF also has an effect on immune function, including measurable physiological changes such as an increase in mast cells,

Elevate Your Health

which indicates the body's allergic response and inflammatory conditions.

▶ Lai (2014) shows the link between ELF and neurological effects, while studies have also found that mobile and cordless phone exposure causes an increased risk of brain tumours and/or acoustic neuromas, especially if you use it on only one side of your head.

Since the time between exposure and diagnosis of cancer for most brain tumours is between fifteen and twenty-five years, and mobile phones have only been in widespread usage for about ten to fifteen years, you can see how this would be a problem.

▶ There are other effects such as headaches and depression, especially for children and adolescents, since ELF suppresses melatonin production, which causes difficulties with sleeping. Burch's study on mobile phone usage shows that twenty-five minutes of use a day has a significant impact on melatonin production.

▶ Stress is another factor. There's a release of stress proteins that occurs due to the presence of an environmental toxin, such as EMF. Concentration and memory problems can be a result from ELF and RF. In humans, there's a change in brainwave activity, and there's been a proven effect on animals.

▶ It may surprise you that tinnitus is a symptom shared by EHS sufferers.

▶ There's also the subject of male and female infertility. Please never keep your phone in your pocket, close to any sex organs. For women, never wear your phone in your bra. Mobile radiation at standby levels have been shown to affect the female animal reproductive system, which decreases ovarian development.

I would encourage all mothers to limit their cell phone use during pregnancy and take necessary precautions. Divan, et al., in 2008, found that children had more of a chance of having emotional problems, hyperactivity and general conduct problems, and thus more peer problems.

▶ According to Lai and Singh, (2004), EMF low strength fields can damage DNA, which causes replication errors, breaks DNA strands and impedes protein synthesis. These symptoms are sometimes misdiagnosed as Chronic Fatigue Syndrome.

### What can people do if they think they're sensitive to EMFs?

Assess your environment in the home, workplace and especially where you sleep. If you have electromagnetic hypersensitivity, you'll need to reduce your long-term exposures to levels well below average to relieve your symptoms. If you don't have EHS, you may need do no more than become better aware of the issue. A great idea is to get a specialist to undertake a site inspection.

### What levels are considered safe?

That's really difficult to say. If your understanding of safety is that there's no effect on humans, particularly children, I don't think anyone can say that. People with EHS are sensitive to EMF at much, much lower levels than the current guidelines. The BioInitiative Report recommends levels lower than 1mG. Building Biology Evaluation Guidelines for sleeping areas are more conservative, with a recommendation level of below 0.2mG.

### What steps would you suggest for using modern technology while remaining mindful of its potential impact on health?

Most health and safety initiatives have a control hierarchy that generally covers the same topics.

1. Eliminate, where possible, the source of the field.

2. Substitute the item for a one less harmful, such as:

   • battery-operated appliances like alarm clocks.

   • wired/cabled phones and routers.

3. Administer: education, housekeeping, job rotation and maintenance.

4. Engineer: use materials that reduce EMF by shielding.

5. Personal Protective Equipment (PPE) is the last resort. However, some serious EHS sufferers may need to use this option.

## What other factors should people consider?

People who are particularly vulnerable, such as babies and young children, or those sensitive to EMF, may need a higher level of protection when exposure can't be reduced to levels of safety or comfort.

Children have more brain fluid and a thinner skull, relative to adults. They're more susceptible to EMFs. A twelve-month-old child absorbs nearly twice as much radiation per kilogram than an adult.

I shall leave you with something thought-provoking. If you want further proof that as an individual you need to be the master of your destiny, ask a mobile phone manufacturer for evidence their insurers will cover them for lawsuits regarding the health hazards produced by their products.

Probably the largest re-insurance company in the world, Swiss Re-insurance, backs up the insurance industry for claims they may not cover, but Swiss has refused to accept liability for claims concerning mobile phones and health effects. In 1997, nearly twenty years ago, it advised the insurance industry of this issue. Perhaps the insurance industry is anticipating something nobody's yet realised. Maybe when phone companies are sued and will have to fold because they're not insured, it will all come to light. I wonder.

> "The world is a dangerous place to live; not because of the people who are evil, but because of the people who don't do anything about it."
> ~ *Albert Einstein*

### When does a person need to hire a professional consultant?

If you're not sure of your exposure, a professional consultant can conduct a comprehensive EMF survey and provide advice. They will have expertise in the reduction of EMFs, including shielding refrigerators, electrical panels, and whole rooms where necessary. I incorporate this within a comprehensive health and safety survey of your home and deal with such issues of concern as indoor air pollution and use of chemicals.

### What are the 3 DEs?

I've developed a mechanism that's consistent with the control hierarchy.

Steps are based on the 3- DEs:

1. *Determine* where the exposure is likely to be coming from.

   Go around your home and examine your use of electricity. Do you turn devices off that are located near the wall when they're not in use? If not, consider this as a minimum practice and one that saves you money. An added benefit to your pocket as well as your health.

Survey your home and list your likely exposure sources. Don't forget to look in your external environment for powerlines and mobile phone towers.

Call a family meeting to discuss what you've learnt here. Try to change your family's attitude to electricity, not by scaring them into returning to the pre-industrial age and forcing them not to use electricity, but by using it more wisely with concern for everyone's health.

2.  *Decrease* your exposure by distancing yourself from the source and/or limiting the time period of exposure. *Example:* when the microwave is in use, don't stand next to it. You're being exposed to a high EMF. Find something to do at the far side of the kitchen or even vacate the kitchen for a time.

    Remember the inverse square rule, which in effect is *more distance=less EMF.*

    If you have an unavoidable and long task, think about ways to minimise your exposure by changing the activity.

    *Example:* The EMF exposure from a long task on a laptop computer could be reduced by primarily using your computer's battery power and recharging the battery while you're having a break from screen time or doing other tasks such as off-screen reading. Move away from the computer while it's charging.

3.  *Defend* yourself with a shield.

    If you're sensitive to EMF, there are ways you can reduce your exposure by putting up protective barriers between you and the EMF source. There are a range of options you might consider.

Some work well and others less so.

In conjunction with other means of reducing exposure, these methods can be fairly successful for some people. There are a few engineering measures that incur expense, so it's wise to seek the advice of a professional before you make a purchase. Inappropriate shielding can be expensive and may not help or even make the problem worse. A professional survey may indicate cost-effective ways of reducing exposure to acceptable levels.

Practical strategies may include having an electrician make changes to your electrical wiring, such as:

- having all of the twenty-four hour electrical essentials, like the fridge, and perhaps cable TV, on an independent circuit. All other circuits can be turned off at the switchboard at night or available via demand switches

- bundling cables to cut down on the EMF produced or shielding the wiring

- relocating the wiring in the wall cavities, especially in bedrooms, to run down through from the ceiling, thus distancing EMF from people

You should relocate appliances to areas well away from the living room or bedrooms where your family spends much of their time. It's worth considering, but remember that internal walls are no barrier to EMF. Special paint can be used to protect surfaces. On windows, shielding film can help with radio frequencies. But again, seek the services of a professional, as depending on your circumstances an off the shelf or retail solution may not be the cheapest or most effective. Sometimes it can make the problem worse. Without the professional survey you may not even know.

### What other tips do you have for reducing exposure?

▶ At a minimum, turn off your Wi-Fi at night. Wherever possible, use hard-wired internet connections. If you're near your neighbours, consider turning the Wi-Fi off when you leave your home unattended. Your pets will thank you.

▶ If you can see more than your own Wi-Fi with a strong signal on your computer, you're being exposed to your neighbours' Wi-Fi and vice versa. Talk to your neighbours about your concerns in a positive, non-confrontational manner. See if they're willing to change their practice as well. This will probably be mutually beneficial.

▶ Try to do without a microwave. If you can't, at least distance yourself from it during its operation.

▶ DECT cordless phones use the same frequency as mobile phones, so long conversations should be avoided. They also emit EMF continuously from their base station. See if you can replace your DECT phone with a hard-wired phone.

▶ Avoid digital (DECT) baby monitors, due to their proximity to the child and that they pulse bursts of microwave radiation a hundred times every second. Talkback models similarly are not recommended for the same reason.

▶ Take care regarding underfloor heating. It can be a high EMF emitter. If you have babies or toddlers, they will be getting the worst of it.

▶ Pay close attention regarding the sitting of high EMF emitters like electricity meters, smart meters, fridges and microwaves. If there's a bedroom in the next room, it's equally as dangerous. If this isn't practical, move the bed to the other side of the room.

- Be careful with extension cables, particularly if they're close to furniture you use frequently.

- Laptops should be on battery power and not placed on your lap. Also use a hardwired Ethernet connection with your wireless router turned off.

- Try to eliminate/reduce the electricity-consuming items from the bedroom. Don't keep a DECT phone or AC-powered alarm clock within two metres of the bed. This includes two metres into an adjoining room as well. Metal spring mattresses and metal bed frames can produce an electromagnetic field if they are, or have been, close to an electric field.

- Electric blankets should be avoided, as even when switched off and not heating, they can produce a field.

- The transformers in gaming consoles, like Play Station and Xbox, can create a large electric and electromagnetic field. Wireless hand controllers can give off high radiofrequencies similar to a mobile phone. They're often used in the lap, but you should avoid doing this and remain at a safe distance from the transformer. Switch off consoles when not in use.

- You also shouldn't use a tablet in your lap, especially in the case of children. Operate it in flight mode whenever possible, as constant pulsing occurs, even when the internet is not in use.

- Women shouldn't carry mobile phones in their bra, and nobody should carry mobile phones in their pockets, close to reproductive and other organs.

### Do you have any final thoughts to share?

I started by saying I wanted to let you know the risks. I hope you feel I've given you enough information to at least have a basic understanding and awareness. If you were unaware about EMF and have become interested, do some research about it. Here's some further reading, if you so desire:

The BioInitiative Working Party Report, 2012

*Overpowered: The Dangers of Electromagnetic Radiation (EMF) and What You Can Do about It*, Martin Blank, PhD, 2014

*The Force: Living Safely in a World of Electromagnetic Pollution*, Lyn McLean, 2011

A list of references used in this chapter can be provided by the author upon request.

Ultimately, I must leave it up to you as to how you choose to safeguard you and your family. Go ahead and evaluate the evidence and weigh the risks of inaction, and if you're convinced, implement your own measures based on the precautionary principle.

Share what you've learnt with a friend. They might not be aware of the risks.

In workplaces, there are occupational health and safety standards that dictate which action can be taken. At home, there's only *you*.

> "The world is a dangerous place to live; not because of the people who are evil, but because of the people who don't do anything about it."
>
> ~ Albert Einstein

To discover more about how Russell can help you *Elevate Your Health*, visit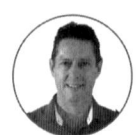

www.elevate-books.com/health

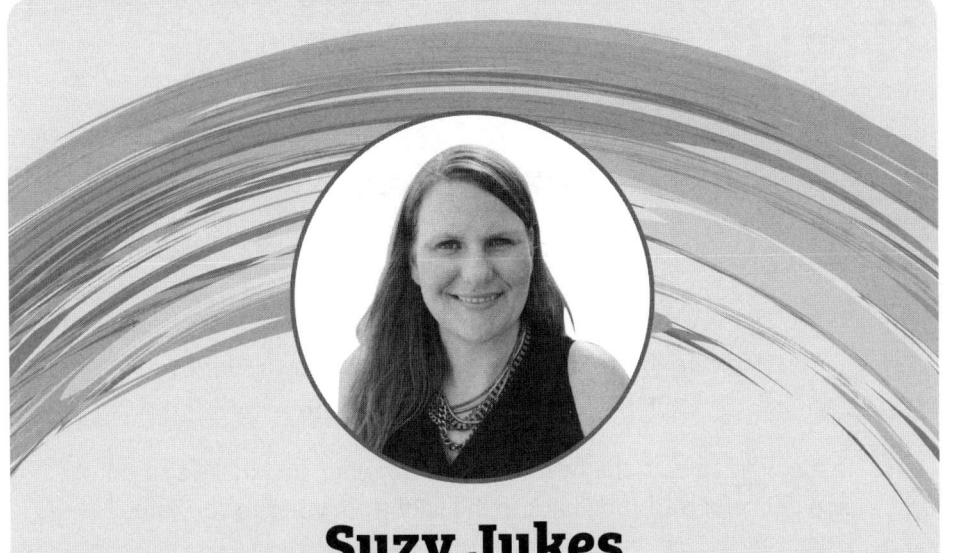

# Suzy Jukes

## Mojo Mentor

Suzy is a powerful healer, creator and visionary leader.

She has a degree in Business Logistics, and has worked in management roles at world-class events, including The Melbourne 2006 Commonwealth Games and the Asian Games in Qatar.

Suzy has completed a PHD: Programs for Heart-Centered Difference-Makers, with Authentic Education. She's a qualified international coach and sacred sexuality educator who's done extensive professional training in healing, tantra, personal development and meditation.

Suzy specialises in sexual healing. She uses concepts from traditional Western medicine, combined with the latest scientific research and ancient shamanic and alternative therapies, to help people around the world heal themselves.

# Suzy Jukes

## Mojo Mentor

I dedicate this to my mother, who passed away during
the final stages of writing this book.

"To the woman with the heart of gold. May your soul make a smooth
and peaceful transition back to the light from whence you came."

I love you, Mum.
RIP Dorothy aka Grandma Butterfly
4th August 2016

### What's been your best manifestation?

The coolest manifestations that came true would be having a million
dollars in my bank account and a mortgage-free home. Let me go back
to the beginning. A little over ten years ago, I knew a woman named
Doreen Virtue. She's an amazing lady who helps people connect with
those who have passed on, as well as get in touch with their own
intuition.

My mum really wanted to go to Doreen's course in Sydney, so I bought
her a ticket. It was on her wish list of what she wanted to do before
she passed. Mum went to a free event in Melbourne and was really
inspired to get her book signed by Doreen. At the lunch break she
went and got her book signed, and Doreen said to her, "Oh, you're
very clear." She was referring to Mum's aura, or her energy. Mum just
said thank you, got her book signed and sat back down.

Then Doreen came back on stage and said there was a guy who'd been
nagging her, because he wanted to speak. He was a soul who'd passed
over. She asked the crowd if it was okay to let him speak, and they

agreed. His name was Gary, and she asked if there was anyone who'd lost someone with that name. A few people put up their hand, but then she clarified that he'd committed suicide.

It turned out to be for my mum, since Gary was my brother Tony's best mate. His nickname was Bart, like Bart Simpson, and my brother had tried to stop him from going through with it, but unfortunately Gary decided to take his own life anyway. The message coming through to Doreen was to let my brother know everything was okay, and it wasn't his fault, because he was going to do it anyway. Gary also said to please tell his parents he was on the other side. The message for my mum was to thank her for helping him cross over to the light and that my mum's purpose on this planet is to help people's souls cross over.

Gary said he was on the other side helping other young souls cross over as well. At the end, the guy who organises tickets asked my mum to come to Doreen's course in Sydney and wanted to give her a complimentary ticket. My mum explained I'd already paid for her to go, but Doreen insisted on giving us a refund. My mum came home and offered me my money back, and I said if this was for real I wanted to see it for myself. So I took the free ticket, and we went off to Sydney. The course was amazing. I've now done it three times.

The first time I went, Doreen did this abundance meditation. There was a roomful of people in the Darling Harbour Convention Centre, and after the meditation she said, "Okay, I want you to visualise whatever it is you want in your life." I remember just seeing the inside of a house. It was white and lit up and had Cathedral ceilings. All I remember is the inside of this house and that I wanted a mortgage-free home, because I was with a partner who was about to go bankrupt. I would get stressed every week, since we didn't have enough money to pay for the mortgage and all of the other bills.

Then Doreen said, "Okay, now visualise how much money you want in your bank account." And I thought, *I'm not greedy. I'll just have a million dollars, thanks.* So I saw myself going to an ATM machine and taking out like a hundred dollars and then getting the little ATM statement that showed I had a million dollars. Fast forward seven years later, about five years ago now, and I'd saved up money for a deposit to buy my own house.

I was looking at places to live. My dad flew in, sat me down in his hotel room and told me I'd handled myself pretty well, and he was proud of me. He was referring to me leaving my partner, because I'd realised I needed to make some changes. He also talked about how I forgive people and was on the right path. He said he didn't want to see me struggle, so he decided to give me my inheritance early and wanted to buy me a home.

He told me what my budget was, and I just started looking for a house. I walked into the place I'm living in now and right away noticed the cathedral ceilings. It's exactly the house I saw in the visualisation. I was so grateful. The night before the closing was stressful as I waited for the settlement to take place. The money hadn't gone into my account yet, so I couldn't sleep. I rang up the bank, and the automated voice recording told me I had one million dollars in my account.

I called again, and it said the same thing. The next day, just like in my visualization, I went to the ATM and withdrew a hundred dollars. I still have the ATM slip in my drawer that shows the million dollar balance. When I went into the bank to tell them what happened, they told me they'd accidentally hit the send button twice. It's like in Monopoly, when you get the card that reads, *Bank error in your favour.* Only in the game, you get to keep the money and spend it on more property.

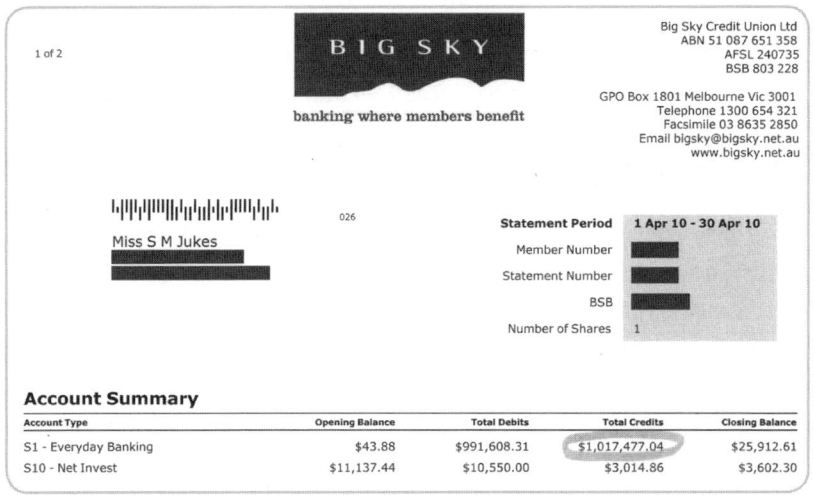

I was impressed that the abundance meditation was so powerful that both circumstances I'd visualised happened on exactly the same day and realised it was too much of a coincidence for me. I decided to look deeper and asked myself how I was different from everyone else. Like, how did this happen? What had I done differently?

### Did this experience lead you down the path you're on now with Mojo Mentor?

Totally. These events were massive turning points in my life. Firstly, at the course in Sydney I learned how to access and tap into my intuition and what I liked to call my *higher intelligence*. Of course, this wasn't easy, and still to this day I don't always follow my intuition, so it leads me into all sorts of trouble.

It's fortunate that I have a great sense of humour, so I can laugh at myself. Like anything, intuition is a muscle that needs exercise. A lot of exercise. Get slack, and you start listening to that other voice in your head, the ego, which consists of made-up beliefs you formed when you were about seven years old. This is not an ideal age for forming an identity, that's for sure. So I was fascinated by the topic of intuition. I began to take action by watching videos and reading books on other Hay House authors similar to Doreen Virtue. I was forced to eat a bit of humble pie. My former disbelief turned around when I realised there were so many experts, all with the same type of message.

You really can alter your life through your beliefs and heal your own body. The more I looked, the more evidence I found to support that spirituality is real, and the best part of it is that science is now starting to catch on and back it all up. There's Neuro-plasticity and metaphysics, espoused by scientists like Bruce Lipton in his book, *Biology of Belief*, and Gregg Braddon's, *The Divine Matrix* is all about heart intelligence. I was blown away.

I left my partner a few years after the course, as our life paths were just headed in different directions, and I continued on my quest to find answers. I've spent the past ten years researching these greats and have countless mind maps from breaking it all apart. You could say I was stuck in *analysis paralysis*. I was also too scared to give up my fulltime logistics job and just go for it.

But I finally did. I think I'm needed in the sexual health and education arena, because my background makes me unique. In fact I cringe when at the start of some small spiritual courses I attend, the facilitator says, "Now, let's talk logistics. Okay, so toilets are down the back at the end of the hall, and we should have lunch around one pm," because they just don't get it.

Logistics is defined as the complex organisation of a detailed operation. Take the bread you toast for breakfast each morning. Logistics consists of the processes and systems that start from growing and harvesting the grain in the field to it winding up on your table. That's why I believe I can help people join the dots quickly when it comes to the delicate topic of sex. I can break it down into bite-sized chunks, so you can easily apply it to your own life.

### Do you think mindset is important?

Everyone goes on about mindset being your best friend when it comes to healing, success and transformation, and it's true. Mindset is also key when it comes to manifesting. Belief is king. It's unfortunate that when people go to manifestation courses they want instant results, and they don't apply their knowledge. They give up before their dreams come true.

I started researching spirituality and manifesting, because I'd spent years thinking my mum was away with the fairies, when it turns out I was the one with my head in the sand. Like the saying goes, *It's what you don't know that matters most*. Well, take it from me, when I landed one million dollars in my bank account and a mortgage-free home per my crystal-clear visions, that was enough to make me take action.

My logical brain was fixated on understanding the science of how this happened. So I made a promise to myself that when I worked out logically the reason behind my extraordinary manifestation success and how I could explain it simply, I'd share it with the world, because, I'm just a regular woman who used to think that spirituality was all a little bit *woo-woo*. I was convinced I could recreate the same success. More importantly, I wanted to get the message across that if I could do it, so could anybody.

What I realised was that it wasn't all just about mindset. The piece of the puzzle missing from manifestation and most healing, transformation and success courses lies within your sexual *mojo*. In other words, everyone has some mojo inside of them. Some power that seems almost otherworldly. It's *all* about Mind-Body-Mojo. Why is it missing? Because most people have shame around their sexuality, and no one wants to talk about it. That's where I fit into the picture. I'm not a doctor, so anything I say is not medical advice. What I can share are my beliefs and the research of doctors. Take on board what you choose and leave the rest.

I believe you can heal your body. That thoughts, feelings and beliefs affect your physiological health in more ways than you can imagine. Why do I believe this? Because I've healed myself of some minor ailments. I've also followed closely the work of Dr Lissa Rankin, a medical doctor who cured herself of a disease. She's moved from Western medicine to now help people understand how powerful the mind is and that there's actual scientific data that proves people can heal themselves. In her New York Times bestseller, *Mind Over Medicine*, Dr. Rankin refers to the Spontaneous Remissions Project that documents over 3,500 cases of people with seemingly incurable diseases healing themselves.

Dr Rankin states that Western medicine definitely has its place, and rightly so, but the mind can cure the body. She states that a combination of positive beliefs and the support of the *right healthcare practitioner*, along with a positive approach from the client, can transform the body in ways that science is only just now beginning to understand. She explains that you wouldn't take a pill from a bottle with a skull and crossbones on it, but every negative thought poisons your body. She also says that every time you feel optimistic and have the support of your community or the will to get in touch with your life purpose and spiritual self, you're healing your body.

### Do people need to come in and see you, or can your method be done over the phone and Skype?

Most of my healing and mentoring work these days is done over the phone.

### What is your major life lesson?

Aside from how we can heal ourselves, especially from sexually related issues, my other major lesson is that life rewards action, and with determination, belief and practise you can achieve anything. After my manifestation came true, I understood the science behind it and continued to practise my skills and enhance my technique, which led to more and more remarkable occurrences.

I also practiced my mojo manifesting skills for charity. For two years running, I wore a school dress every day in October to raise money to send girls back to school in Sierra Lione, West Africa, because a girl over there is more likely to get sexually assaulted than attend high school. See my website for details on some of the crazy stunts I pulled in a school dress, like skydiving and stand-up comedy. Over two years I raised over $17,000 just from my family and friends on Facebook.

### What is The Mojo Mentor?

The Mojo Mentor is all about empowering you to get your mojo back in full force and have an extraordinary sex life, even if you're single. The best things in life are free. Everybody deserves the right to a healthy and fulfilling sex life. I help people bust through their shame around sexuality and use their sexual desire for self-healing, pleasure and transformation.

The Mojo Mentor is also about getting people to start talking about their sexuality. I'm passionate about providing a safe space where people can open up and communicate about what's going on for them around their sex lives.

I've worked with a large number of men who are married and say that they haven't had sex for months and sometimes years. I ask them one simple question: have you actually sat down and had an authentic and real conversation about this with your partner? Most say no and rattle off some excuse about why they haven't. Therein lies the problem. Sexual desire is the greatest of all mind stimuli, and you can't help but think about it because we are all sexual beings, but nobody is talking about it.

The result is repressed emotions around sexuality, which eventually leads to physical ailments. In men, it leads to decreased sexual performance and loss of sensitivity from trying to take care of themselves on their own. For women, repressing emotions around sexuality can also lead to impotence, mood swings and a feeling of letting their partner down by not wanting sex. I know women who actually withhold sex from their partner as a way of punishing them. It's time for people to stop feeling shame around their sexuality and to open up and communicate about what's going on for them in that area.

This program is about healing the mind, body and mojo. It's about owning both your light and shadow and using your sexual fantasies and desires, the greatest of all mind stimuli, for self-healing and transformation.

I want you to listen to your body. I want to inspire you to stop living in shame and start getting your mojo on, so you can express yourself as the sexual being you are.

I believe your spirit is your mojo. My dream is for there to be more love in the world. I want people to start tapping into their inner essence and choose love over fear. Openly communicate your desires and wants, and feel safe in doing so. Then just go for it. Live in the moment, and don't look back.

In essence, the mission behind The Mojo Mentor is to create more love in the world.

I'm really passionate about helping people tap into their own sexual energy and using it to create success. I believe it's the most powerful energy there is, and a lot of people don't realise it. As a result, they get frustrated. For instance, if you've been single for a long time and want to become sexually active, understand that you could be channelling this energy into whatever it is you want to create in the world.

**When you say sexual energy, do you just mean the desire to have sex?**

Yes, in a way. Of all human desires, sexual desire is the most powerful. The mind really responds to it. But that's only where it starts. Sexual energy is the emotion. If you break down the word, it's energy in motion. It's like a little furnace inside you're not tapping into.

At a young age, I happened to walk in on a man while he was self-pleasuring himself. I wound up exploring this behaviour by giving myself intimate pleasure at a time when my mum and dad separated, and my mum went overseas for many years. During these times, I would think about getting good grades at school and other issues I was having, and it enabled me to manifest some really cool things into my life.

**How do people find out about you? This is such a specific specialty.**

Go to my website www.themojomentor.com and suzyjkes.com.

**There's a rich history in what you do, right?**

There's a book entitled *Think and Grow Rich* by Napoleon Hill, and it was written back in the 1930s. I refer my clients to chapter eleven. What it says is if a man can use his sexual energy for something other than active sex itself, they can create genius. So that's basically what I want people to do. Use their sexual energy to help them create whatever they want or just have a better life for themselves, whatever way or shape it takes.

My dad had a website back in 1987, when the Internet had only first come out. His was one of three websites dealing with the G-spot, and it was the first educational one.

When I discovered tantra and became a sex education teacher, I learnt so much. For example, I didn't know women could have over seven different types of orgasms. But I have to admit, I found a few tantra teachers a little bit too yogie/hippie/spiritual. That's why I take a more logical approach. Also, I didn't feel they were abundant in their way of thinking.

Don't get me wrong. My mum is as spiritual as they come, and I'm into spirituality as well, but the general public isn't, and so trying to mix sexuality with spirituality is only going to work for some of the population. I want to create a global movement. The Mojo Movement, if you will, where people can freely talk about sexuality without feeling like it's some taboo topic. I like to be unique, so all of my teachings are backed up with solid science. My logistical mindset has broken all of the concepts down into bite-sized pieces. In this way you can easily join the dots and get down to the core of your sexual issues to heal yourself in a simple, easy and fun way. I feel that's what sets me apart.

What I've uncovered from talking to men, is that it's all about their self-confidence and frustration. A lot of my clients are married but having issues in the bedroom. Just look at the divorce rate. I'm sure a lot of the cases are because there are issues around one partner wanting more sex than the other or maybe they have some kind of dysfunction. It really affects people in so many different areas of their life. It's the same for women. They're not standing up and asking for what they want, because they have low self-confidence. It all goes back to sexual energy or mojo.

**Is there one particular message you want to share with the world?**

Yes. I want people to use their mojo to help them create a better life.

**What legacy do you want to leave?**

I want to help people transform their mojo into success. You know... *sexcess*!! Don't be ashamed of your sexuality. Speak up and communicate more about something that's sacred and beautiful and such a powerful healing and transformational tool.

**When you're travelling, what do you never leave home without?**

A genuine nephrite Tantric Jade Egg! Ladies, please visit my website for more details on this extremely powerful healing and manifesting tool.

**What are the steps to mojo mastery?**

In this game of life, you get to choose your own adventure. Every decision is based on love or fear. Thoughts are either empowering or disempowering. Beliefs will either leave you feeling fulfilled or like a failure. Ultimately, you must decide to either play small with a minimum impact result or play full out for maximum gains.

There are ten steps to Mojo mastery. This list of questions will give you a basic understanding as to what the Mojo Mastery System is all about.

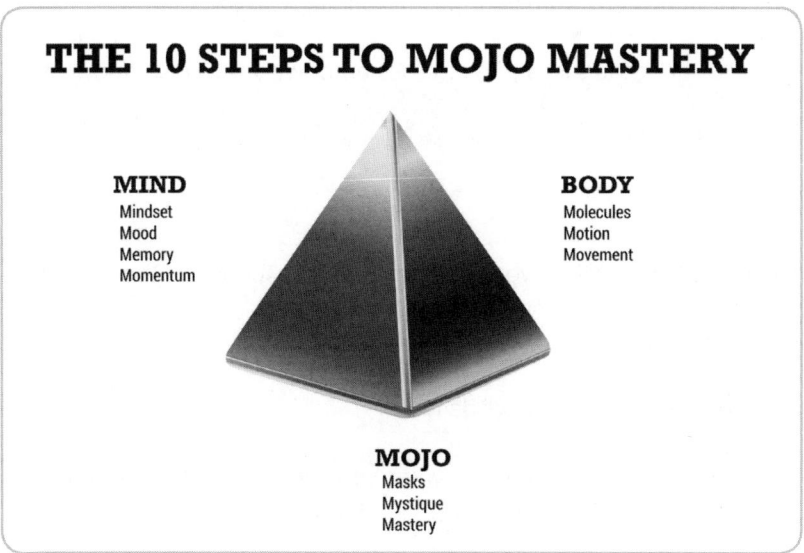

1. MINDSET

How does your mindset shape your reality? To work this out, ask yourself the following questions:

▶ Are your beliefs based on LOVE or FEAR?

▶ Are your thoughts based on LOVE or FEAR?

▶ Are your feelings based on LOVE or FEAR?

## 2. MOOD

▶ How are you showing up in the world?

▶ What is your current state of play?

▶ Are your actions based in love or fear?

## 3. MEMORY

▶ What incident from your past is holding you back?

▶ Are your thoughts and memories empowering or disempowering?

▶ Are they based in love or fear?

## 4. MOLECULES

Think about the cells in your body and their response to the following:

▶ How do you react to situations that happen to and around you?

▶ Do you watch the news daily?

▶ If so, how do you react to what you see, particularly news about acts of terror? Do you respond in fear?

▶ If you choose not to watch the news, is it because you want to remain in a state of love?

## 5. MOTION

This section is all about your energy levels.

▸ Do you have stuck emotions in your body?

▸ Do you have repressed emotions in your body from past traumas that haven't healed properly?

▸ Does your body react to fear? Does it sway back and forth like a pendulum in motion, depressed sometimes, and elated at others, or are you good at remaining centred and balanced when life throws curveballs your way?

## 6. MOVEMENT

▸ How well do you adapt to change in your life?

▸ Does your body move with grace and flow?

▸ Is your body operating in a state of love or fear?

## 7. MASKS

▸ What masks are you wearing in the world?

▸ How would you feel if there was a camera in your house filming live to YouTube twenty-four hours a day?

▸ What sections would you delete?

▸ Does this thought fill you with love or fear?

## 8. MOMENTUM

▸ Are you ready to move forward fearlessly?

▸ Are you willing to take action and go for the gold?

## 9. MYSTIQUE

▸ What unique gift do you bring to the table?

▸ What do you have that lights you up and when you share it, lights up the life of others? For instance, do you have a contagious laugh that fills a room? Do you love to laugh? What makes you shine like the star that you are?

## 10. MASTERY

▸ Do you have the discipline, courage and commitment to make a real difference in the world?

▸ Are you ready to live in a world full of love, compassion, understanding and acceptance?

### *Who are your inspiring role models?*

Comedians! I love how they can so easily look at the bright side of life and laugh at themselves. I often say my life is like a Seinfeld series. That's a show literally about nothing, just the lives of some ordinary people, which is what makes it so funny. I like to look for the humour in my life as well. My branding is based around *Austin Powers* and his lost mojo for a reason. After all, he's the one who brought the term mojo back into our world.

But my most inspirational person is Jim Carey. This is a man who manifested ten million dollars for his role in *Dumb and Dumber* using some of the same principles I teach as part of the Mojo Mastery System.

Thank you to Jim Carrey for your most eloquent words to sum up this chapter.

> *"I've often said that I wished people could realize all their dreams of wealth and fame, so they could see that it's not where you'll find your sense of completion...I can tell you from experience, the effect you have on others is the most valuable currency there is... Everything you gain in life will rot and fall apart, and all that will be left of you is what was in your heart...Fear is going to be a player in your life, but you get to decide how much. You can spend your whole life imagining ghosts, worrying about your pathway to the future, but all there will ever be is what's happening here, and the decisions we make in this moment, which are based in either love or fear. So many of us choose our path out of fear disguised as practicality. What we really want seems impossibly out of reach and ridiculous to expect, so we never dare to ask the universe for it. I'm saying, I'm the proof that you can ask the universe for it — please! ....as far as I can tell, it's just about letting the universe know what you want and working toward it while letting go of how it might come to pass...You are ready and able to do beautiful things in this world and...you will only ever have two choices: love or fear. Choose love, and don't ever let fear turn you against your playful heart."*

**When you moved out of logistics and into healing, were there fears you had to overcome around leaving a secure job and going out on your own?**

A hundred percent. It was one of the scariest things I've ever had to do. It was terrifying to give up a good income, but I figured following my heart and living my love was much more important than money, so I'm so glad I did. I love my job so much. I make a difference in people's lives every day, and that makes me feel so great.

**If you were speaking to your younger self, what advice would you give her?**

Get off your butt and take action. Stop listening to what other people say, and just go for it, because you're living in a box if you're listening to everybody else. Take the chance. Whilst you might cop the flack, don't worry about it. Follow your heart, and you'll be fine.

Stay positive, no matter what anybody says. It's okay if you're single. Just use the time to help create what you're out there to do.

**What do you think is the secret behind your success? What drives you?**

My clients tell me it's because I really do care. I'm serving people because I genuinely want to help them. This is my passion.

 To discover more about how Suzy can help you *Elevate Your Health*, visit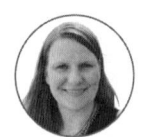

www.elevate-books.com/health

# Afterword

While you were reading these people's inspiring stories, did you notice something? All of their life experiences were for a purpose, bringing them closer to their goals, relationships and especially the message they were meant to share with the world.

The last page is a blank canvas for you to write the next chapter of your own story about elevating your health and inspiring others. Every day is a brand-new opportunity to be the author of your destiny.

# Next Steps

To support you on your journey to *Elevate Your Health*, we recommend you take advantage of these resources:

## 🖥 7 Day Transformation Program

Learn ONE powerful 'Elevate Process' you can use immediately to improve Your Relationships, Health, Finances, Mindset and any other area of your life.

To join this 7-day transformation online program, simply go to: www.elevate-books.com/you

## 👥 Connect with the Authors

To discover more about the authors and what they have to teach you, and bonus gifts they are offering visit:
www.elevate-books.com/health

## 🎤 Subscribe to our Podcast

If you'd like to hear the go-to interviews from the authors and be re-inspired, check out: www.elevate-books.com/podcast

## 🌐 Visit the Website

To find out more about the Elevate book series, visit: www.elevate-books.com